PRESCHOOLERS & KINDERGARTNERS
MOVING & LEARNING

Other Redleaf Press Books by Rae Pica

Toddlers Moving & Learning

Early Elementary Children Moving & Learning

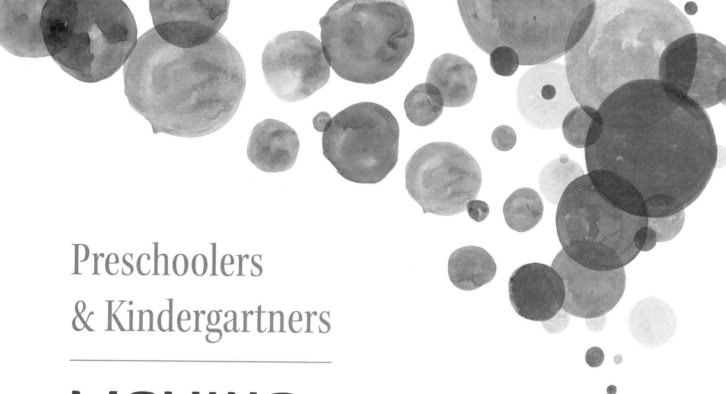

Preschoolers
& Kindergartners

MOVING & LEARNING

RAE PICA

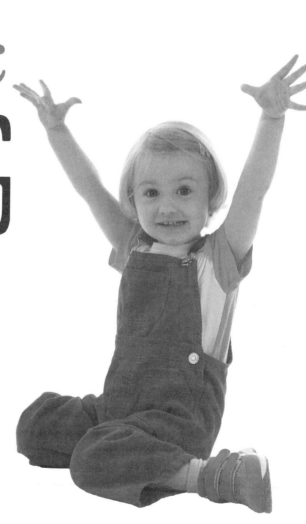

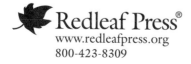

Redleaf Press®
www.redleafpress.org
800-423-8309

Published by Redleaf Press
10 Yorkton Court
St. Paul, MN 55117
www.redleafpress.org

First edition 2014
Cover design by Ryan Scheife, Mayfly Design
Cover artwork composed from images: (empty room) ssstep/iStockphoto; (watercolor circles abstract and colored spots) crisserbug/iStockphoto; (child gestures) tompet80/iStockphoto
Interior design by Ryan Scheife, Mayfly Design
Typeset in Kepler MM
Interior illustrations by Chris Wold Dyrud
Printed in the United States of America
21 20 19 18 17 16 15 14   1 2 3 4 5 6 7 8

Guidelines on pages 11–12 are from *Active Start: A Statement of Physical Activity Guidelines for Children from Birth to Age 5*, 2nd ed., by the American Alliance for Health, Physical Education, Recreation and Dance (AAHPERD) (Reston, VA: AAHPERD, 2009). Reprinted with permission.

Excerpts on page 13 are from *Developmentally Appropriate Practice in Early Childhood Programs Serving Children from Birth through Age 8*, a position statement by National Association for the Education of Young Children (NAEYC). Copyright © 2009 NAEYC. www.naeyc.org/files/naeyc/file/positions/PSDAP.pdf. Reprinted with permission.

Excerpts on pages 12–13 are from *NAEYC Standards for Early Childhood Professional Preparation Programs*, a position statement by NAEYC. Copyright © 2009 NAEYC. http://www.naeyc.org/files/naeyc/file/positions /ProfPrepStandards09.pdf. Reprinted with permission.

Library of Congress Cataloging-in-Publication Data
Pica, Rae, 1953-
 [Preschoolers and kindergartners moving and learning]
 Preschoolers & kindergartners moving & learning / Rae Pica.
   pages cm
  Summary: "Physical education is a critical part of the early childhood curriculum, and it helps children develop lifelong love for fitness and healthy habits. This movement program includes standards-based lesson plans with many fun activities" — Provided by publisher.
  Includes bibliographical references.
  ISBN 978-1-60554-268-3
  1. Movement education—Study and teaching (Elementary) 2. Early childhood education—Activity programs. 3. Physical fitness for children. I. Title.
 GV452.P5197 2014
 372.86'8—dc23
                    2013031260

Printed on acid-free paper

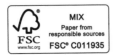

*The three books in the Moving & Learning series
are dedicated to my "angel," Fredrick Davis.
He knows why.*

Contents

Acknowledgments

I couldn't be happier that the Moving & Learning series is finding a home at Redleaf Press. It's become clear to me that this is where these books belong. I'd like to thank Kyra Ostendorf and David Heath for the warm welcome, with extra-special thanks to David for being a fabulous editor. Working with you was such a pleasure!

I'm forever grateful to Richard Gardzina for the original music that accompanies these curriculum packages. He is a remarkable composer, and what I especially love about what he created here is that he never considered it "children's" music. Instead, he set out to compose and perform the best music he could.

Special thanks to the children and teachers with whom I've worked over the years—those on whom I "practiced" and those who've embraced the "movement message" at my presentations. Your enthusiasm, along with your expressions of appreciation over the years, has kept me going!

Deep appreciation to my mom, whose pride in me warms my heart.

Activity Chart

Lesson	Body-Parts Activities	Nonlocomotor Activities	Locomotor Activities	Movement-Element Activities
1	Heads, Shoulders, Knees, and Toes	Let's Bend	Let's Walk	Exploring Up and Down
2	Show Me	Let's Stretch	Walking Along Again	Big and Little
3	My Fingers	Bending and Stretching	Let's Run	Bridges and Tunnels
4	See My Hands	Let's Shake	Creepy-Crawly	Making Shapes
5	See My Face	Let's Sway	Let's Jump	Pop Goes the Weasel
6	Simon Says	Let's Bounce	Rabbits and 'Roos	Moving Backward
7	The Body Song	Exploring Bending and Stretching	Moving Like Animals	Moving Slow/Moving Fast
8	Mirror Game	Let's Turn	Marching Band	Exploring Body and Spatial Directions
9	Hands-Hands-Hands	Let's Sit	Let's Leap	Moving Softly/Moving Loudly
10	A Face Has Many Roles in Life	Let's Push and Pull	Let's Gallop	Marching Slow/Marching Fast
11	Switcheroo!	Let's Strike	Follow the Leader	High and Low
12	Body-Part Relationships	Let's Lift	Shadow Game	Robots and Astronauts
13	Traveling Body Parts	Let's Swing	Locomotion I	Exploring Force
14	Exploring Right and Left	Let's Twist	The Tightrope	Exploring Movement Elements
15	Exploring Weight Placement	In My Own Space	Let's Hop	Staccato/Legato
16	Counting Body Parts	Imitating Movement	Let's Roll	Getting Fast/Getting Slow
17	Arms in Motion	Let's Focus	Let's Slide	Getting Louder/Getting Softer
18	Legs in Motion	Pass a Movement	Let's Skip	Common Meters
19	Body-Halves Opposition	Dodging in Place	Locomotion II	Different Strokes
20	Left Side/Right Side	Combining Nonlocomotor Skills	Combining Locomotor Skills	Exploring Space

Curriculum Connectors Chart

Lesson	Activity	Art	Language Arts	Math	Music	Science	Social Studies	Page
1	Heads, Shoulders, Knees, and Toes		X		X	X		32
1	Let's Bend			X		X		33
1	Let's Walk		X		X	X	X	35
1	Exploring Up and Down	X		X		X		37
2	Show Me					X		40
2	Let's Stretch			X		X		41
2	Walking Along Again				X		X	43
2	Big and Little	X	X	X				44
3	My Fingers		X	X	X	X		46
3	Bending and Stretching	X		X		X		48
3	Let's Run				X		X	50
3	Bridges and Tunnels	X	X	X	X		X	52
4	See My Hands					X	X	54
4	Let's Shake	X	X	X	X	X		56
4	Creepy-Crawly		X			X		59
4	Making Shapes	X	X	X				61
5	See My Face					X	X	64
5	Let's Sway				X	X	X	65
5	Let's Jump		X			X		67
5	Pop Goes the Weasel		X		X			69
6	Simon Says		X		X	X		72
6	Let's Bounce	X		X		X		74
6	Rabbits and 'Roos			X	X	X		75
6	Moving Backward	X	X	X			X	76
7	The Body Song		X		X	X		78
7	Exploring Bending and Stretching		X	X		X		79
7	Moving Like Animals		X			X		80
7	Moving Slow/Moving Fast			X	X		X	82
8	Mirror Game	X	X				X	86
8	Let's Turn					X		87
8	Marching Band		X	X	X		X	89
8	Exploring Body and Spatial Directions	X	X				X	90
9	Hands-Hands-Hands		X		X		X	94
9	Let's Sit		X	X				96

(CONTINUED ON NEXT PAGE)

Curriculum Connectors Chart (continued)

Lesson	Activity	Art	Language Arts	Math	Music	Science	Social Studies	Page
9	Let's Leap		X	X		X		97
9	Moving Softly/Moving Loudly		X	X	X	X		98
10	A Face Has Many Roles in Life		X		X		X	100
10	Let's Push and Pull					X		101
10	Let's Gallop		X		X	X		103
10	Marching Slow/Marching Fast			X	X		X	104
11	Switcheroo!					X	X	106
11	Let's Strike			X		X	X	107
11	Follow the Leader	X	X		X			109
11	High and Low	X	X	X	X			111
12	Body-Part Relationships	X		X		X		114
12	Let's Lift			X		X	X	115
12	Shadow Game	X	X			X	X	117
12	Robots and Astronauts				X	X	X	118
13	Traveling Body Parts	X		X		X		120
13	Let's Swing					X		122
13	Locomotion I		X		X		X	124
13	Exploring Force			X		X		126
14	Exploring Right and Left	X		X		X		128
14	Let's Twist				X	X	X	129
14	The Tightrope		X			X	X	130
14	Exploring Movement Elements	X	X	X		X		132
15	Exploring Weight Placement					X		136
15	In My Own Space		X			X		137
15	Let's Hop					X		138
15	Staccato/Legato		X		X		X	139
16	Counting Body Parts			X		X		142
16	Imitating Movement	X	X	X				144
16	Let's Roll					X	X	145
16	Getting Fast/Getting Slow		X	X	X			146
17	Arms in Motion	X	X				X	148
17	Let's Focus					X	X	150
17	Let's Slide				X		X	151
17	Getting Louder/Getting Softer	X	X	X	X		X	152
18	Legs in Motion		X					156

(CONTINUED ON NEXT PAGE)

Curriculum Connectors Chart (continued)

Lesson	Activity	Art	Language Arts	Math	Music	Science	Social Studies	Page
18	Pass a Movement			X			X	157
18	Let's Skip		X		X			158
18	Common Meters			X	X			160
19	Body-Halves Opposition		X			X		164
19	Dodging in Place					X	X	165
19	Locomotion II		X		X			166
19	Different Strokes		X		X		X	167
20	Left Side/Right Side		X			X		170
20	Combining Nonlocomotor Skills		X					171
20	Combining Locomotor Skills		X					172
20	Exploring Space	X	X	X	X			173

Song List

Title	Length	Page
"Walking Along"	1:41	35
"Walking Along Again"	2:21	43
"The Track Meet"	1:22	50
"Shake It High/Shake It Low"	2:58	56
"The Swaying Song"	2:02	65
"Pop Goes the Weasel"	1:24	69
"Rabbits and 'Roos"	1:44	75
"The Body Song"	2:21	78
"Moving Slow/Moving Fast"	2:44	82
"Marching Band"	2:55	89
"Hands-Hands-Hands"	2:46	94
"Moving Softly/Moving Loudly"	2:47	98
"A Face Has Many Roles in Life"	3:19	100
"Giddy-Up"	1:39	103
"Marching Slow/Marching Fast"	2:24	104
"High and Low"	1:50	111
"Robots and Astronauts"	3:19	118
"Locomotion I"	3:28	124
"Twisting"	2:10	129
"Staccato/Legato"	3:13	139
"Getting Fast/Getting Slow"	2:26	146
"Getting Louder/Getting Softer"	2:31	152
"Skipping Song"	1:09	158
"Common Meters"	3:59	160
"Locomotion II"	4:47	166
"Different Strokes"	3:45	167
"Exploring Space"	3:32	173

Introduction

Welcome to the Moving & Learning family! The movement program in your hands, *Preschoolers & Kindergartners*, is being used in schools, child care settings, recreation centers, and gymnastic centers throughout the United States and in several other countries.

The program consists of twenty lesson plans, with four activities per plan (not including extensions). Each lesson is intended to take approximately forty-five minutes to complete. (Alternatives are discussed later, under "Implementing the Program.") The twenty lessons and their activities have been arranged in a developmental progression, from least to most challenging, with each lesson plan consisting of one body-parts activity, one nonlocomotor activity, one locomotor skill experience, and one activity exploring an element of movement.

The lessons begin with simple body-part identification, which is the basis of any movement experience. The lessons also begin with the simplest locomotor skills (movements that transport the body from one place to another) of walking and running. (Technically, crawling and creeping are the simplest, but the exploration of these skills has been incorporated later, in order to promote a feeling of "maturity" among the children.) The simplest nonlocomotor skills (movements performed while remaining in one place) of bending and stretching are also found in early lessons, along with the simplest movement elements of space and shape.

If you start at the beginning and progress in a logical, developmental manner, you can expect greater success from children who are encouraged to build upon their earlier successes as stepping stones. You can also expect greater *response* from them as well. The idea is to make the children feel good about experiencing movement—by starting slowly and providing them with frequent opportunities to experience success. If children are asked to respond to challenges that they could not possibly be comfortable with or are not prepared for, the result is intimidation and a lot of blank stares. No wonder—that would be comparable to asking a fledgling ballet student to perform a perfectly executed *tour en l'air* (turn in the air) without first acquainting her or him with the basic balletic skills!

Children need opportunities to explore movement on their own, to find and use their own personal rhythms, so not all of the activities in this book are accompanied by music. However, children do love music—and it does contribute much to movement experiences—so it is included wherever it can make a contribution to the learning experience. The songs that are part of this program are almost entirely original, having been written specifically for the activities they accompany. (Activities using music have been marked with a musical note: ♪.) The songs make it possible for you to add the joy and energy of music to movement experiences without the effort of having to first *locate* appropriate music. They also make it possible for the children to better understand such abstract concepts as slow and fast, light and heavy, and bound and free. These songs expose the children to both electronic and acoustic instruments and to as many musical elements (for example, tempo, volume, and so on) as I could manage to include. Variety is what I believe in, and variety is what this curriculum offers the children, and you!

Every activity in *Preschoolers & Kindergartners* includes some simple questions to help you evaluate whether or not the children are meeting the activity's objectives. The Curriculum Connectors feature points out ways in which the activity correlates, or can be made to correlate, with other content areas.

While it is my firm belief that the body is the most important piece of equipment in movement experiences, I realize that using actual equipment can add another dimension to—and increase the challenge of—an activity. So, where appropriate, I have included a section called Adding Equipment, offering suggestions for the use of hoops, scarves, streamers, and other props generally available in early childhood classrooms.

Benefits of Moving & Learning

Movement experiences in general—and this curriculum specifically—have many benefits for children. They exercise the whole body, including the mind, and not just the muscles; they create a love of movement that should develop into a lifetime desire for physical fitness; and their success-oriented philosophy provides numerous opportunities for learning, participating, and enjoying. The following are some of their more specific benefits.

Physical Development

Perhaps the simplest and most important reason children should be allowed and encouraged to move is to develop movement skills.

Although it is commonly believed children automatically acquire motor skills as their bodies develop, maturation only means that children will be able to execute most movement skills at a low performance level. Continuous practice and instruction are needed if the performance level and movement repertoire are to increase (Gallahue and Cleland Donnelly 2003). In other words, once a child is able to creep and walk, gross-motor skills should be taught—just as other abilities are taught. Furthermore, special attention should be paid to children demonstrating gross-motor delays, as such delays will not simply disappear over time.

As Linda Carson explains, families and teachers "would not advocate learning to read or communicate by having their children enter a 'gross cognitive area' where children could engage in self-selected 'reading play' with a variety of books" (2001, 9). Similarly, engaging in unplanned, self-selected physical activities—or even a movement learning center—is not enough for young children to gain movement skills.

Why does the development of motor skills matter, when not every child will go on to become an athlete or a dancer? It matters because children who feel confident in their movement skills are likely to continue moving throughout their lives. And that's significant because of the many health problems that can be attributed to sedentary living.

Although children love to move—and adults tend to think of them as constantly being in motion—children today are leading much more sedentary lives than did their predecessors. According to Nielsen research, "Younger children age 2–5 log close to 25 hours of TV time each week, more than 4.5 hours watching their favorite DVDs, about 1.5 hours viewing DVR offerings, more than an hour competing at video games and 45 minutes with the VCR" (McDonough 2009). In fact, watching television is the predominant sedentary behavior in children, second only to sleeping (Kaur et al. 2003). The advent of computers and video games has also contributed to the decline in activity. A study from the Kaiser Family Foundation determined that children ages eight to eighteen are spending more than seven and a half hours a day with electronic devices (Lewin 2010)—the same number of hours some people spend at full-time jobs.

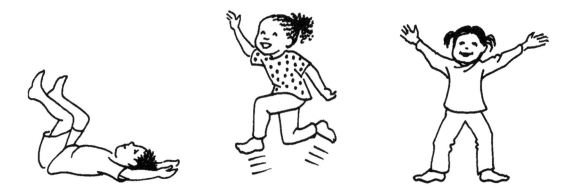

According to Bar-Or et al., there is one consistent observation that stands out among the studies of energy expenditures in young children: children under the age of seven seem to expend about 20 to 30 percent less energy in physical activity than the level recommended by the World Health Organization (1998). The Children's Activity and Movement in Preschools Study (CHAMPS) determined that children enrolled in preschools were "engaged in moderate to vigorous physical activity (MVPA) during only 3.4 percent of the preschool day" (NIEER 2010). Pate et al. observed two thousand children and found that "children attending preschools were engaged in MVPA during only 2.6% of observation intervals. During over 85% of intervals, children were engaged in either very light activity or sedentary behaviors" (2008, 443).

Considered together, these factors provide cause for concern regarding children's fitness levels. Statistics indicate that 40 percent of five- to eight-year-olds show at least one heart disease risk factor, including hypertension and obesity. The latter, which is on the rise, particularly among children, has been linked to television viewing (Bar-Or et al. 1998). A Canadian study determined that the blood vessels of obese children have a stiffness normally seen in much older adults who have cardiovascular disease (Science Daily 2010). Furthermore, the Centers for Disease Control and Prevention (CDC) estimates that American children born in the year 2000 face a one-in-three chance of developing type 2 diabetes, previously known as adult-onset diabetes because it was rarely seen in children (2008).

A developmentally appropriate movement curriculum, such as *Preschoolers & Kindergartners*, can give children the practice and instruction necessary to refine their movement skills and expand their movement vocabularies. Moreover, with *Preschoolers & Kindergartners*, the children have the opportunity to frequently experience success, which makes movement pleasurable for them. Thus they are more likely to become (and stay!) physically fit.

Social/Emotional Development

Marianne Frostig, in her classic book *Movement Education: Theory and Practice*, says,

> Movement education can help a child to adjust socially and emotionally because it can provide him with successful experiences and permit interrelationships with other children in groups and with a partner. Movement education requires that a child be aware of others in [activities] in which he shares space . . . ; he has to take turns and to cooperate. He thus develops social awareness and achieves satisfaction through peer relationships and group play. (1970, 26)

This book provides opportunities for successful experiences, and it permits interrelationships with other children. Even before the children are asked to work cooperatively with partners and groups, they must be aware of others around them, adjusting their movement patterns to avoid collisions. Of course, any time children work in pairs or in groups, as they will have an opportunity to do with this curriculum, they are learning lessons in cooperation and consideration.

This book also offers a blend of teacher-directed activities and a creative problem-solving approach to instruction. The latter lends itself to success by allowing children to respond to challenges at their own developmental levels and rates. This approach increases children's self-confidence, and thus their self-esteem, as they see their choices being accepted and praised. According to Muska Mosston and Sara Ashworth, two important results of problem solving are the "development of patience with peers and the enhancement of respect for other people's ideas" (1990, 259).

The development of *empathy* is also promoted through exposure to certain social issues that will, hopefully, make positive impressions in your preschoolers' and kindergartners' young and open minds. For example, to physically imitate the movements and characteristics of a variety of animals is to imagine what it is like to *be* those animals. Those of us who wish to see children raised with a healthy respect and compassion for all the world's creatures can certainly hope that once our children have imagined what it is like to be the animals, they will never be able to imagine a world *without* them.

Cognitive Development

It has been said that joy is the most powerful of all mental stimuli. For young children, movement is certainly joyous. Beyond that, however, studies of how young children learn have proven that they especially acquire knowledge experientially—through play, experimentation, exploration, and discovery.

For example, when children move over, under, around, through, beside, and near objects and others, they better grasp the meaning of these prepositions and geometry concepts. When they perform a "slow walk" or skip "lightly," adjectives and adverbs become much more than abstract ideas. When they're given the opportunity to physically demonstrate such action words as *stomp*, *pounce*, *stalk*, or *slither*—or descriptive words such as *smooth*, *strong*, *gentle*, or

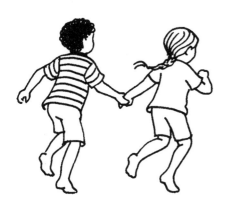 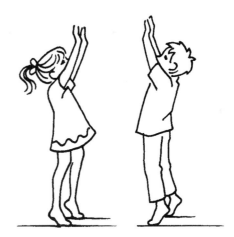

enormous—word comprehension is immediate and long lasting. The words are used and learned *in context*, as opposed to being a mere collection of letters. This is what promotes emergent literacy and a love of language.

Similarly, if children take on high, low, wide, and narrow body shapes, they'll have a much greater understanding of these quantitative concepts—and opposites—than do children who are merely presented with the words and their definitions. When they act out the lyrics to "Ten in the Bed" ("There were five in the bed, and the little one said, 'Roll over'..."), they can *see* that five minus one leaves four. The same understanding—and fascination—results when children have personal experience with such scientific concepts as gravity, flotation, evaporation, magnetics, balance and stability, and action and reaction.

Additionally, learning by doing creates more neural networks in the brain and throughout the body, making the entire body a tool for learning (Hannaford 2005). There is a growing body of research determining that physical activity activates the brain much more so than doing seatwork. While sitting increases fatigue and reduces concentration, moderate- to vigorous-intensity movement feeds oxygen, water, and glucose to the brain, optimizing its performance.

Beyond providing an opportunity for children to "feed" their brain and to learn by doing, *Preschoolers & Kindergartners* contributes to cognitive development in the following ways:

- These movement experiences offer numerous opportunities for the children to deal with the concepts of space and shape. Thus they will be better able to deal with abstract thought. Language, numbers, and the alphabet are all abstractions, so this is very necessary preparation.

- Directionality and spatial awareness are critical to reading and writing abilities.
- By using a problem-solving method of instruction with the children, you will also be enhancing their problem-solving capabilities. They are going to discover there will always be more than one way to solve any problem or to meet any challenge.
- The children will experience cross-lateral movement, which helps children cross the body's midline and activates both hemispheres of the brain in a balanced way. Because such movements involve both of the eyes, ears, hands, and feet, as well as core muscles on both sides of the body, they activate both hemispheres and all four lobes of the brain. This means cognitive functioning is heightened and learning becomes easier (Hannaford 2005).
- Body image influences a child's emotional health, learning ability, and intellectual performance.

Creative Development

Can you imagine a world without creativity and self-expression—not just in the arts, but in science, business and industry, education, and life itself?

Can you honestly say you do not find some creativity in each and every preschooler or kindergartner you work with—or that you do not know at least one adult who has lost the ability to express himself or herself, creatively or otherwise? Where does creativity go from the time we are preschoolers and kindergartners to the time we become adults? Is that loss of potential a result of a society and an educational system that fail to emphasize creativity and individuality?

Why is creativity important? There are a lot of reasons. However, for young children, creativity means there is no one *right* answer. This enhances their sense of mastery, which in turn promotes their self-esteem and helps them realize they can indeed have some effect on their environment.

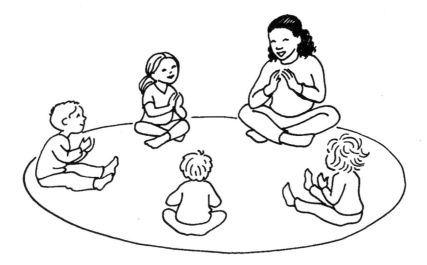

Teresa M. Amabile reported that the key personality traits of highly creative people, if not naturally occurring, can be developed in childhood. These traits include

- self-discipline about work;
- perseverance when frustrated;
- independence;
- tolerance for unclear situations;
- nonconformity to society's stereotypes;
- ability to wait for rewards;
- self-motivation to do excellent work; and
- a willingness to take risks.
  (1992)

According to Mary Mayesky,

> Adults who work with young children are in an especially crucial position
> to foster each child's creativity. In the day-to-day experiences in early child-
> hood settings, as young children actively explore their world, adults' attitudes
> clearly transmit their feelings to the child. A child who meets with unques-
> tionable acceptance of her unique approach to the world will feel safe in
> expressing her creativity, whatever the activity or situation. (2009, 24)

Preschoolers & Kindergartners encourages children to find their *own* ways of responding to challenges, to be individuals, and to *imagine*. When you meet their uniqueness with "unquestionable acceptance," the children will be better

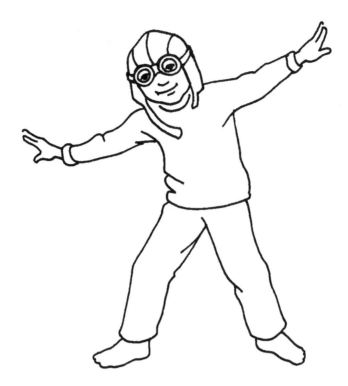

equipped later in their lives to imagine solutions to problems they face, to feel empathy, and to plan futures that are full and satisfying.

As Margaret Newell H'Doubler so aptly writes in her classic book, *The Dance and Its Place in Education,*

> as every child has a right to a box of crayons and certain instruction in the fundamental principles of the art of drawing, whether there is any chance of his ever becoming a great artist or not, so every child has a right to know how to obtain control of his body so that he may use it, to the limit of his abilities, for the expression of his reactions to life. (1925, 33)

Benefits to Children with Special Needs

All of the benefits previously cited can be applied to children with special needs. Additionally, coordination, listening skills, conceptual learning, and expressive ability are just a few of the areas enhanced through regular participation—at whatever level possible—in movement experiences.

Perhaps of greatest importance, however, is the contribution that movement experiences can make toward the special child's self-concept. Often children with disabilities fail to form a complete body image due to exclusion from physical activity. Similarly, because they do not necessarily perform the same way other children do, they develop a distorted body image (Gallahue and Cleland Donnelly 2003). Identifying and moving various body parts can "help the child discover how each body part fits into the whole schema of a human body. This enables the child to explore body boundaries and define his/her body image" (Samuelson 1981, 53). Achieving regular success in movement activities will contribute greatly to the child's confidence—perhaps offering for the first time an opportunity to feel good about himself or herself.

Another unique opportunity derived from the movement program is the chance to be part of a group. As the child's self-concept becomes more developed, he is better able to relate to others. As the child's movements and ideas are regularly accepted and valued, he receives greater acceptance from his peers. Becoming part of a group—making contributions, taking turns, following rules—has the additional benefit of enhancing social skills.

Meeting Standards

In today's educational climate, meeting standards is a consideration for all education professionals, including those in early childhood. Movement experiences in general, and those in *Preschoolers & Kindergartners* specifically, can address multiple standards outlined by the American Alliance for Health, Physical Education, Recreation and Dance (AAHPERD) and the National Association for the Education of Young Children (NAEYC).

For example, the position of AAHPERD in *Active Start: A Statement of Physical Activity Guidelines for Children from Birth to Age 5* is that "all children from birth to age 5 should engage daily in physical activity that promotes movement skillfulness and foundations of health-related fitness" (AAHPERD 2009, iv). For preschoolers specifically, their guidelines include the following:

1. Preschoolers should accumulate at least 60 minutes of structured physical activity each day.
2. Preschoolers should engage in at least 60 minutes—and up to several hours—of unstructured physical activity each day, and should

not be sedentary for more than 60 minutes at a time, except when sleeping.

3. Preschoolers should be encouraged to develop competence in fundamental motor skills that will serve as the building blocks for future motor skillfulness and physical activity.

4. Preschoolers should have access to indoor and outdoor areas that meet or exceed recommended safety standards for performing large-muscle activities.

5. Caregivers and parents in charge of preschoolers' health and well-being are responsible for understanding the importance of physical activity and for promoting movement skills by providing opportunities for structured and unstructured physical activity. (AAHPERD 2009, 13, 14, 15, 16, and 17)

NAEYC offers *Standards for Early Childhood Professional Preparation Programs*. Among those standards met by *Preschoolers & Kindergartners* are the following:

- Standard 1a: Knowing and understanding young children's characteristics and needs.
- Standard 1b: Knowing and understanding the multiple influences on development and learning.
- Standard 1c: Using developmental knowledge to create healthy, respectful, supportive, and challenging learning environments.
- Standard 3b: Knowing about and using observation, documentation, and other appropriate assessment tools and approaches.
- Standard 4a: Understanding positive relationships and supportive interactions as the foundation of their work with children.
- Standard 4b: Knowing and understanding effective strategies and tools for early education.
- Standard 4c: Using a broad repertoire of developmentally appropriate teaching/learning approaches.
- Standard 5a: Understanding content knowledge and resources in academic disciplines.

- Standard 5b: Knowing and using the central concepts, inquiry tools, and structures of content areas or academic disciplines.
- Standard 5c: Using their own knowledge, appropriate early learning standards, and other resources to design, implement, and evaluate meaningful, challenging curricula for each child.
(2009b, 11, 13, 14, and 16)

NAEYC's position statement *Developmentally Appropriate Practice in Early Childhood Programs Serving Children from Birth through Age 8* specifies that "all the domains of development and learning—physical, social and emotional, and cognitive—are important, and they are closely interrelated. Children's development and learning in one domain influence and are influenced by what takes place in other domains" (2009a, 11). The position statement instructs teachers to "plan curriculum experiences that integrate children's learning *within* and *across* the domains (physical, social, emotional, cognitive) and the disciplines (including language, literacy, mathematics, social studies, science, art, music, physical education, and health)" (2009a, 21).

Implementing the Program

In truth, the term *lesson plan* as it is used in this program is not technically correct; however, a suitable substitute does not seem to exist! Typically, a lesson plan specifies details for teaching *one class period* of a planned learning unit. Nevertheless, it was my intention that teachers would be able to create as many lessons as they want—or deem necessary—from each lesson plan. A great deal of flexibility has been built into this book, so there are probably as many ways to use these lesson plans as there are teachers!

In other words, the fact that there are four activities per plan does not mean that you must complete all four every time you schedule a movement session. Similarly, you should not feel as though you have to use the lesson plans exactly as they are laid out. Although it is important to keep the developmental progression of the activities and their extensions in mind as you go through them, nobody knows the children you teach better than you do. So you should not hesitate to adapt the lesson plans, perhaps abbreviating activities or changing their order, if you feel it is better for your group. If certain activities seem too advanced, feel free to skip them and return to them later; they are offered here simply as possibilities.

You may decide, for instance, that you wish to explore one activity and all of its extensions in a series of movement sessions before moving on to the next activity on the page. Or you may choose to ignore the extensions until you have run through all twenty lesson plans, at which time you can return to Lesson 1 and begin again with the first suggested extension under each activity.

Another option is to add a specific warm-up exercise—a favorite finger-play or song—perhaps, to the beginning of each lesson. Performing the same warm-up all the time can serve to alert your children to the fact that it is movement time. And you can finish with a cooldown of your choice too. For instance, pretending to melt puts closure on the day's lesson by offering children a chance to relax *and* to lower themselves to the floor, where they can await information about what comes next.

No matter how you choose to approach the lesson plans and activities, it is vital that you implement *lots* of repetition. As an early childhood educator, you recognize how important repetition is to young children. Just because a movement activity appears only once in these lesson plans doesn't mean it is intended to be experienced only once! You should repeat activities and even whole lessons as often as necessary to ensure success.

Will you do movement only as part of circle time, or will you schedule longer movement sessions? Will you schedule sessions weekly, daily, or something in between? The following section of the introduction attempts to help you answer some of those questions and provides information you will need to make the best possible use of this program.

Scheduling Movement Experiences

As mentioned earlier, each of the lesson plans in this program consists of four activities and is intended to take approximately forty-five minutes to complete. Whether that holds true for you depends largely upon your particular situation. If you have a very small group of children, for instance, or if you have had to divide a large group in half due to lack of space, you may find that you are able to move through a lesson plan more quickly. If you have more three-year-olds in your class than four- or five-year-olds, you may find that it takes the younger ones longer to complete a single lesson—or that you cannot keep their attention long enough to complete all four activities. Due to the nature of children in general, it is even possible that one lesson will last thirty minutes, the next only twenty minutes, and the following just fifteen!

In other words, you will have to be prepared to play it by ear. However, that should not be a problem. If you have not completed a lesson when your time is up, you can simply pick up where you left off next time. If your class runs short, you can always repeat activities from previous lessons.

My hope, of course, is that you will plan for a daily movement session. If you do movement activities on a daily basis, it is best to use no more than two *Moving & Learning* lesson plans per week, repeating the activities from those lessons throughout the week. Otherwise, the children's senses will be overloaded and focusing will be much more difficult.

Finally, should you wish to adapt the lesson plans, remember that a lesson should include both large and small movements whenever possible. In most cases, this also means that the lesson will consist of both vigorous and not-so-vigorous activities—which you will definitely want to alternate, for your sake as well as the children's.

Creating a Positive Learning Environment

Success is always the goal in a *Moving & Learning* program, so the atmosphere of your class plays an important role. Classroom management must be handled with special care. With so much activity involved, however, maintaining control is not always easy.

Children love to move—and they like to show off and display their abilities—especially to you, so you can use this to your advantage when presenting challenges. If you introduce the challenges with a phrase like "Show me you can" or "Let me see you," the children will want to show you they can. It is a simple technique, but amazingly effective!

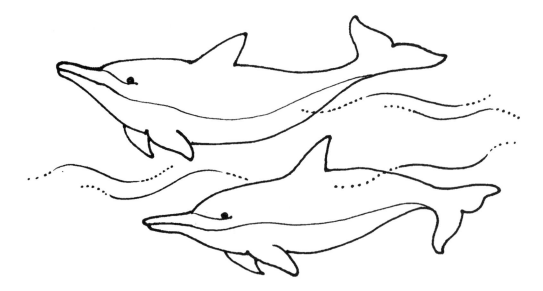

There are fewer behavioral problems when a program is success oriented from the beginning. A child who is experiencing success is less likely to become bored or want to disrupt the class.

There are, however, two important rules you should explain to the children in the beginning and enforce consistently. The first is that there are to be *no collisions*. In fact, there should be no touching unless it happens to be a specific part of an activity. To phrase this positively, you can say, "We will respect one another's space," "We will give each other enough space to move," or "We will always leave enough space for our friends." At the start this may be difficult to enforce, especially with the youngest children—because they generally enjoy colliding with one another! So it is your challenge to make it a goal for the children not to interfere with one another.

You can accomplish this by asking the children to space themselves evenly at the beginning of every movement session. Carpet squares or hoops can help with this. Explain the idea of personal space to them, perhaps by encouraging the children to imagine they are each surrounded by a giant bubble; whether standing still or moving, they should avoid causing any of the bubbles to burst. Another image that works quite successfully is that of dolphins swimming. Children who have seen these creatures in action, either at an aquarium or on television, will be able to relate to the fact that dolphins swim side by side but never get close enough to touch one another. The goal, then, is for the children to behave similarly. Providing pictures of dolphins swimming together could also be helpful.

The second rule that will contribute to a manageable and pleasant environment is that there can be *no noise* (which is different from *no sound*), ensuring that your challenges, directions, and follow-up questions can be heard at all times, with no need for shouting. To phrase this positively, explain that the children are to move as *quietly* as possible. You can accomplish this by establishing a signal that indicates it is time to stop, look, and listen: "Stop, look at me, and listen for what comes next." Choose a signal the children should *watch* for, like two fingers held in the air, or something they must *listen* for—like a hand clap, a strike on a triangle, or three taps on a drum—and make it their "secret code." A whistle is generally not suitable, as it can be heard above a great deal of noise, which means the children will know they can create a ruckus and still hear your signal. (In the same way that a whisper is more effective than a shout, you want a quieter signal that the children have to be *listening* for.) Nor will your voice be effective, as it is heard so often by the children.

If a child still acts out, distracting or endangering other children, ask the child to sit on the sidelines and act as audience. However, give him or her the responsibility of deciding when to rejoin the activities by stating, "When you are ready to join us again, let me know." Whether the child is on the sidelines by request or is simply reluctant to participate, she or he should be allowed to observe only.

In general, as in all matters relating to movement education, a positive attitude is the key. Movement activities should take place in a friendly, encouraging, and fun atmosphere, balanced with some basic ground rules for human behavior. This atmosphere, together with the fact that the children are experiencing success, will ensure that behavioral problems will be minimal.

Suggested Attire

Whenever possible, the children should move in unrestrictive clothing—for obvious reasons. The most important contribution to effective movement is probably the bare foot.

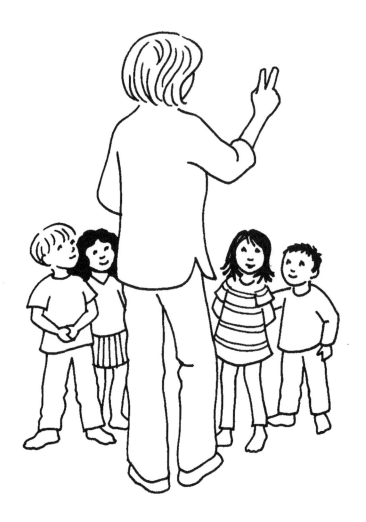

Children have worn sneakers during physical activity for so long now that we seem to have forgotten that the feet do have sentient qualities. They can grip the floor for strength and balance, and the foot consists of different parts (toes, ball, heel) that can be more easily felt and used when bare. Besides, young children feel a natural affinity for the ground, which can be enhanced by stripping away all the barriers between it and the feet.

Of course, sometimes it simply is not possible for the children to perform barefooted, as when a child is wearing tights or health regulations forbid it. If the choice becomes sneakers or stocking feet, then choose the sneakers. It is much too dangerous to move in socks or tights even on a carpet, and sensing how easy it would be to slip will greatly restrict the child's freedom of movement.

Teaching Methods

This book employs the three teaching methods most often used in movement education: *exploration*, the *direct approach*, and *guided discovery*.

EXPLORATION Exploration is developmentally appropriate for young children and should be the teaching method most widely used in movement programs for preschoolers and kindergartners. Because it results in a *variety* of responses to each challenge presented, it is also known as divergent problem solving. For example, a challenge to demonstrate crooked shapes could result in as many different crooked shapes as there are children responding.

This approach to instruction has never been better described than by Elizabeth Halsey and Lorena Porter:

> [Movement exploration] should follow such basic procedures as (1) setting the problem, (2) experimentation by the children, (3) observation and evaluation, (4) additional practice using points gained from evaluation. Answers to the problems, of course, are in movements rather than words. The movements will differ as individual children find the answer valid for each. The teacher does not demonstrate, encourage imitation, nor require any one best answer. Thus the children are not afraid to be different, and the teacher feels free to let them progress in their own way, each at his own rate. The result is a class atmosphere in which imagination has free play; invention becomes active and varied. (1970, 76)

In other words, you will present your children with a challenge (for example, "Show me how tall you can be"), and the children will offer their responses in movement. You can then issue additional challenges to continue with and vary the exploration (*extending* the activity), or you can issue follow-up questions and challenges intended to improve or correct what you have seen (*refining* responses).

Extending exploration is a technique that requires time, patience, and practice by the teacher. When teachers are not yet comfortable with all aspects of exploration, they may hurry from one movement challenge to the next. Not only does this leave the class with too much time and nothing left to do, but it also fails to give children ample experience with the exploration process and with the movements being explored.

In addition to issuing a follow-up to "find another way," you can use the elements of movement (considered adverbs used to modify the skills, which are regarded as verbs) to extend activities. For instance, if the locomotor skill of walking were being explored, there would be a number of choices with regard to *how* to perform the walking: forward, backward, to the side, or possibly in a circle. The element of space is being used here. The walk could be performed with arms or head held in various positions (shape), quickly or slowly (time), strongly or lightly (force), with interruptions (flow), or to altering rhythms (rhythm).

Of course, you must design problems and suggest extensions that are developmentally appropriate and relevant to the subject matter and to the children's lives. You must also provide the encouragement children need to continue producing divergent responses. Encouragement should consist of *neutral* feedback (for example, "I see you're walking in a bent-over shape").

Although you must be careful to accept all responses, there will come a time when you wish to help the children improve, or refine, their solutions. If, for example, you have challenged the children to make themselves as small as possible and some children respond by lying flat on the floor, you should not observe aloud that this response is incorrect. In fact, it is not necessarily incorrect—it is simply another way of looking at things. However, because you want the children to truly experience a small shape, you might use the follow-up question, "Is there a way you can be small in a rounded, or curled, shape?" to encourage a different response. Although you have helped the children improve their responses, individuality is not stifled, as diverse solutions are still possible (for example, some children will make a small rounded shape in a sitting position, some will lie on their backs, others on their sides, and so on).

THE DIRECT APPROACH As children mature, they have to learn to follow directions and to imitate physically what their eyes are seeing (for example, when they must write the letters of the alphabet as seen in a book or on a board). According to Mosston and Ashworth, "Emulating, repeating, copying, and responding to directions seem to be necessary ingredients of the early years" (1990, 45). They cite Simon Says, Follow the Leader, and songs accompanied by unison clapping or movement as examples of "command-style" activities enjoyed by young children. Mirroring and fingerplays are among the other activities that they suggest fit into the same category.

With the direct approach, the teacher makes all or most of the decisions regarding what, how, and when the children are to perform (Gallahue and Cleland Donnelly 2003). This task-oriented approach requires the teacher to provide a brief explanation, often followed by a demonstration, of what is expected. The children then perform accordingly, usually by imitating what was demonstrated.

One advantage of this approach is that it produces immediate results. This, in turn, means you can instantly ascertain if a child is having difficulty following directions or producing the required response. For example, if the class is playing Simon Says and a child repeatedly touches the incorrect body part, you are at once alerted to a potential problem, possibly with hearing, processing information, or simply identifying body parts.

Mosston and Ashworth cite achieving conformity and uniformity as two of the behavior objectives—and perpetuating traditional rituals as one of the subject matter objectives—of the direct approach (1990). For example, if "rituals" like "The Hokey Pokey" are to be performed in a traditional manner, with all the children doing the same thing at the same time, the only expedient way to facilitate these activities is with a direct approach, using demonstration and imitation. Although conformity and uniformity are not conducive to creativity and self-expression, they are necessary to the performance of certain activities. Because such activities are fun for young children and can produce a sense of belonging, they should play a role in the movement program. For preschoolers and kindergartners, however, teacher-directed activities should not play the largest role; that distinction should be given to exploration.

GUIDED DISCOVERY EXTENSIONS Guided discovery extensions, refining responses, and neutral feedback are also elements of the third teaching method employed: guided discovery, which, like exploration, is known as an indirect or child-centered (as opposed to teacher- or task-centered) teaching style.

With guided discovery, also known as convergent problem solving, you will have a specific task or concept in mind (for example, teaching the children to perform a step-hop, or that a wide base of support provides the stablest balance). You then lead the children through a sequence of questions and challenges toward discovery of the task or concept. This process, while still allowing for inventiveness and experimentation, guides the children as they *converge* on the right answer.

One example is a series of questions that leads the children toward discovery of a forward roll. Instead of merely *showing* the children how to perform this skill, you might issue the following challenges:

- Show me an upside-down position with your weight on your hands and feet.
- Show me an upside-down position with your weight on your hands and feet and your tummy facing the floor.
- Show me you can put your bottom in the air.
- Look behind yourself from that position.
- Look between your legs at the ceiling. Try to look at even more of the ceiling.
- Show me you can roll yourself over from that position. Can you do it more than once?

Although guided discovery does take longer than the direct approach, many educators feel its benefits far outweigh the time factor. Among other benefits, with problem solving in general (convergent or divergent), the children are not only learning skills, but are learning *how* to learn. Guided discovery specifically enables children to find the interconnection of steps within a given task.

When using guided discovery with children, it is important to accept all responses—even those considered "incorrect." For example, if you have asked a series of questions designed to ultimately lead to the execution of a forward roll and some children respond with other rolls, these responses must also be recognized and validated. The children can then be given more time to "find another way," or you can continue, asking even more specific questions, until the desired outcome is achieved.

One important tip is that you should never provide the answer (Graham 2008; Mosston and Ashworth 1990). If the answer is given in the beginning, the children cannot discover it on their own, as one cannot discover what one already knows. If the children do not discover the expected solution and you ultimately give the answer anyway, the children will expect this and will be less enthusiastic about exploring possible solutions themselves. Graham also maintains that because "wonder and curiosity are valuable mental processes," there is no harm in concluding a lesson in which the children have yet to discover the solution (2008, 166).

Adapting Activities

Although movement experiences entail an additional challenge for children with special needs, movement education is well suited to these children. Its philosophy and practice lend themselves to inclusion of—and success for—all children. Thus, when incorporating children with special needs into movement activities, you must be sure that your challenges can be met by all of the children.

Keep in mind that every child will be able to respond in some manner. For example, Samuelson explains that the blink of an eye, the inhalation of a breath, and the twitching of fingers are all movements (1981). Thus they can be considered responses to challenges and can even be used for demonstration purposes, with the remaining children being asked to replicate these movements. Not only does this include the child with special needs, but it also places her in what is probably an unfamiliar role—that of leader.

This book, of course, cannot do justice to the vast topic of children with special needs or cover all the different special needs that teachers and caregivers may encounter. However, the following are some guidelines for helping children with physical challenges, hearing impairments, and visual impairments achieve success.

PHYSICAL CHALLENGES In general, the child with physical disabilities should be encouraged to participate at whatever level is possible. A child may have to substitute swaying or nodding the head for more difficult rhythmic responses. If the child cannot hold rhythm instruments, he can wear bells attached to elastics or Velcro placed around his wrists and simply *become* a musical instrument. Children in wheelchairs will have to experience locomotion on wheels rather than on foot—whether propelling themselves or being pushed by a peer.

Cane or crutch tapping can substitute for hand clapping or foot stomping, and upper-body movements can replace lower-body movements.

Movement is typically not a problem for children with hearing impairments unless there is damage to the semicircular canals. If so, the children will have balance problems, which can result in delays in motor ability. Children with such damage should refrain from taking part in potentially dangerous balance activities—for example, climbing or tumbling actions requiring rotation—unless assistance is provided.

AUDITORY CHALLENGES For all children with hearing impairments, the major challenges involved in participating in movement experiences are related to the use of music and the presentation of instructions. You can take a number of steps to help lessen the latter problem. Place children with difficulty hearing in the front of the room. Distractions like background music or others talking should be eliminated. When speaking, you should always face the child with a hearing impairment and avoid covering your mouth. You should also speak in low tones (not low as opposed to loud but low as opposed to high pitched) because children with hearing impairments are better able to hear low-frequency sounds. Flicking the lights off and on is a signal that you can use to instantly get children's attention.

During music activities, remember that although a child may not be able to hear the music, she will be able to feel it. Children with hearing impairments can place their hands on the CD player or the instrument being used to make music to feel the vibrations and establish a rhythm. Lying on a wooden floor often enables children to feel the vibrations with the whole body.

Imitation is another important tool in being able to experience rhythms with and without music. Children with hearing impairments should be encouraged to imitate their peers as they clap hands, stamp feet, march, gallop, and skip.

Finally, movement experiences that meet the needs of children at all levels of ability only need minor modifications to meet the needs of children who are visually challenged. Children with visual limitations tend to rely more heavily on adults than do sighted children and often display hesitation and caution when asked to move. However, they have to their advantage auditory and tactile skills that become increasingly stronger, and these senses can be used to enhance kinesthetic skills.

VISUAL CHALLENGES When working with children with visual impairments, you have a number of methods you can use to help ensure greater success. Children with poor vision should be placed near you so they can see more easily. Holding hands with you or with a responsible partner—or having a partner place his hands on the hips or shoulders of the child with visual problems—are ways of using the tactile and kinesthetic senses to encourage movement and alleviate the fear. You can also use touch to help a child achieve an appropriate shape or position.

To make use of the auditory sense, use verbal cues and clear, succinct descriptions when presenting challenges and when offering feedback. Statements like "You are lifting and lowering your heels to move up and down" have the additional benefit of increasing the child's body awareness. Such statements as "Everyone tilt their head side to side" help the visually impaired child realize that her body is like the other children's.

No matter what special needs a child may have, he or she can be included successfully in most movement activities.

Making Transitions

Whether the children are going on to another content area, to lunch, or home to parents at the end of your movement activities, it is always a good idea to help them wind down a bit before sending them on their way. This is where some relaxation techniques come into play.

You may be surprised to learn that relaxation plays other important roles in movement experiences than just offering rest. Relaxation prepares children for slow or sustained movement, which requires greater control than fast movement. Being relaxed also provides children with the opportunity to experience motionlessness, giving more meaning, in contrast, to movement. Tension control can also help children learn better, as stress has a negative impact on learning. Additionally, if you use imagery to promote relaxation, you will be enhancing the

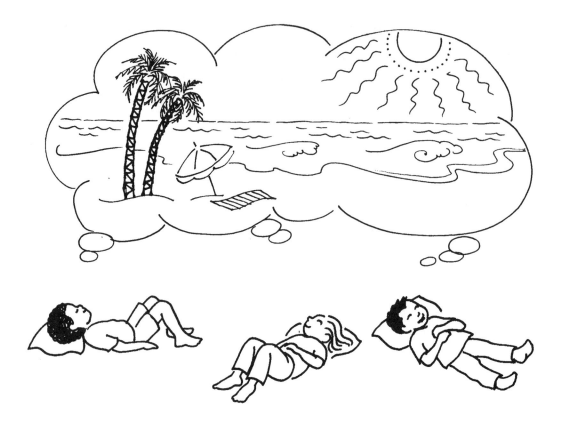

children's ability to imagine. If you use music, you will be exposing the children to the world of quiet, serene music. The following are some specific suggestions.

IMAGERY What comes to mind when you think of rag dolls, limp noodles, melting ice cubes, or soggy dishrags? Relaxation! Ask the children to pretend to be one of these objects, and just watch those muscles relax. Or paint a picture in their minds: Ask them to lie on the floor, imagining they are floating on a cloud or at the beach. For the latter, talk to them (softly!) about the warmth of the sun, the cool breeze, and the gentle sounds of the waves and the gulls circling overhead; and do not be surprised if a few of them drop off to sleep.

SLEEPING CONTEST If you have a particularly competitive group of children, you might find that a sleeping contest works best of all. Ask them to show you who in the class can sleep the soundest (without snoring!), and just watch as they drop to the floor! Of course, there can be no one winner, so you will have to congratulate them all on being the best sleeping class you have ever seen.

Music There are many soothing pieces to choose from, whether with vocals or without—including classical music from the distant past (Mozart, Bach, and Chopin wrote some wonderfully soothing pieces) as well as New Age music, lullabies, or some of the many children's recordings made specifically for "quiet times."

Teaching Hints

The following suggestions are offered to help you facilitate movement experiences as smoothly as possible:

- Always familiarize yourself with a lesson or activity, and particularly with a song *before* trying it with the children.

- When an activity calls for music, the lesson plan will specify this with a musical note (♪) and indicate which song on the accompanying CD is to be used. The Song List will help you find the song you need.

- Discuss new or unfamiliar words or images from songs or poems with the children prior to the activity.

- Introduce each activity to the children ("Now we're going to explore *up* and *down*").

- Always be sure children are both familiar and comfortable with an activity before trying its extensions.

- The lesson plans leave plenty of room for your personality and imagination. Please feel free to use them!

Preschoolers and Kindergartners: Developmental Considerations

The following is some information concerning the characteristics and development of children ages three to six years. Some of these facts are ones you are already aware of and serve here as reminders. Together with the others they will give you a better idea of what you can expect from your children as you begin this program.

- The younger the preschoolers, the more time they will need to organize themselves as a group—a fact you should keep in mind if planning movement sessions as short as fifteen minutes.
- Forty-five minutes is generally the greatest length of time you can expect to keep preschoolers and kindergartners interested and involved in movement activities.
- Preschoolers run into objects and one another because depth perception is a learned ability. Therefore, their paths must be kept clear, and the children must be allowed enough time to change directions.
- When verbal instructions are given, the initial motor response of five-year-olds will be toward the sound of your voice.
- Four-year-olds generally require the highest level of physical activity.
- Hand dominance is generally established by five years of age.
- The development of gross (or large-muscle) motor skills will occur according to each child's individual timetable. By three years of age, however, children usually have good large-muscle control. Fundamental movement abilities are usually present by five years of age; by the age of six, children are able to perform most locomotor skills in a mature pattern (at a well-developed level).
- Preschoolers and kindergartners may tire suddenly, but they recover quickly.

Here are some other general milestones that normally take place by certain ages.

By age three, a child should be able to do the following:

- walk on tiptoe for ten feet
- balance on one foot for five seconds

By age four, a child should be able to do the following:

- walk on tiptoe for long distances
- balance on tiptoes and on one foot for approximately five seconds
- walk a four-inch low balance beam

- execute seven to nine hops on the preferred foot
- gallop with a steady rhythm (still with preferred foot leading)
- perform four or more successive slides in the same direction

By age four and a half, a child should be able to do the following:

- balance on one foot for approximately ten seconds
- walk backward toe to heel
- hop on the nonpreferred foot
- gallop rhythmically and steadily with either foot leading
- perform a slide in either direction

By age five, a child should be able to do the following:

- walk a two-inch balance beam
- hop on one foot for long distances, holding the free foot to the rear and using arms for balance
- maintain a skip over approximately twenty to thirty feet, although usually with an uneven (short-long) rhythm

By age five and a half, a child should be able to do the following:

- skip steadily, although probably still with an uneven rhythm
- demonstrate steadiness and consistent rhythm in sliding

It is critical that children develop efficient movement patterns during early childhood; otherwise they will find it more and more difficult to do so with every year they age. Your role, therefore, is an important one. Although you will primarily be using exploration as a teaching method, you must still be aware of how *well* the children are performing movement tasks.

However, you will notice that, like the children, the skills listed here are also developmental. Just because developmental guidelines indicate that a child of four should be able to walk on tiptoe for long distances, you must not expect your four-year-olds—if they can do it at all—to perform this task flawlessly. Your children will first perform each new skill in imperfect, individual ways; you should be concerned only if a child shows no progress toward mastering it after faithfully practicing the skill for a long period of time.

Caroline Sinclair writes that

the preschooler up to the age of five is very busy learning new ways to move and practicing those he already knows. He can be helped best by being provided opportunity, motivation, encouragement, and a certain degree of protection, and by being allowed full rein for his creativity and discovery. (1973, 64)

LESSON 1

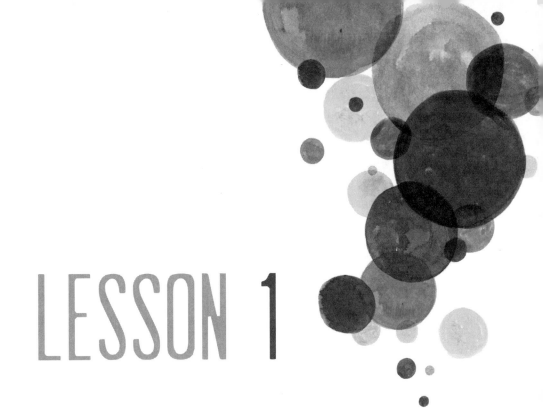

Heads, Shoulders, Knees, and Toes

Ask the children to touch their heads, shoulders, knees, and toes as you call out the names of these parts. Once the children are experiencing success with this, reverse—and mix up—the order of the body parts.

Extending the Activity: Vary the tempo at which you call out the body parts, or start out slowly and gradually accelerate (*time*). Add dramatic pauses—long and short—so the children are not sure when you will call out a body part (*flow*). Call out the body parts in a steady *rhythm*, perhaps challenging the children to add a clap between each touch.

Observation and Evaluation: Can the child identify the appropriate body parts? Does the child demonstrate listening skills?

Adding Equipment: Children can touch rhythm sticks, instead of their hands, to the body parts. If you are calling out the body parts rhythmically, the children can click their sticks together instead of clapping hands.

Curriculum Connectors: Body-part identification is an important introductory concept for young children, falling under the theme of "My Body" and the content area of *science*. Listening skills are a part of both *language arts* and *music*.

Let's Bend

Have the children stand and experiment with bending forward, backward, and to both sides. Then issue the following challenges:

- Touch your knees and straighten.
- Touch your toes with your knees bent (to avoid strain on the lower back) and straighten up very slowly.
- Touch your toes and straighten up more quickly.
- Touch your toes and straighten up only halfway.

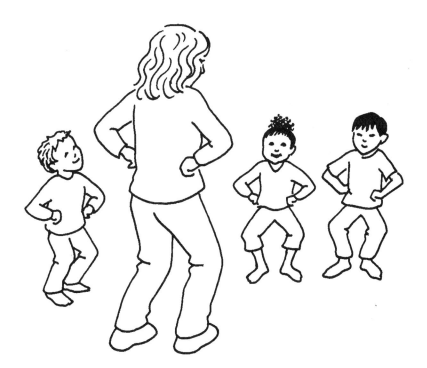

Extending the Activity: Follow this up by asking the children to experiment with bending the waist, arms, and legs while kneeling, crouching, sitting, and lying on backs, stomachs, and sides (*space* and *shape*). Challenge them to bend different body parts as though in slow motion, or in "fast-forward" (*time*). Can they bend various body parts as though against a lot of pressure, or as though they were weightless (*force*)? Add more challenging body parts, like fingers, wrists, and ankles.

Observation and Evaluation: Is the child able to bend the applicable body parts and in the appropriate directions? Does the child seem to understand the concept of bending?

Adding Equipment: Invite the children to bend various body parts while balancing a beanbag on the body part being bent, or on another, such as the top of the head.

Curriculum Connectors: To make *mathematics* a part of the activity, challenge the children to count the number of ways each part can bend. Which part can bend the most ways? The fewest? Experimenting with the limitations and capabilities of body parts constitutes *science*. Incorporating balance, by adding the beanbags, brings an additional science concept into the exploration.

Let's Walk

 "Walking Along" (Length 1:41)—CD Track 1

This activity provides an excellent opportunity for you to observe the children's strengths and weaknesses with regard to posture and alignment, weight distribution, and use of body parts—while the children simply have fun walking. Observing closely, have the children walk in the following ways:

- freely (while being straight and tall)
- in place ("Show me you can make your knees go higher. Show me you can do it faster.")
- forward ("Show me you can you walk slower.")
- on tiptoe ("Show me you can you make yourself even taller.")
- on heels (briefly)
- very slowly; very quickly
- with tiny steps; with giant steps
- very lightly; very strongly
- walk-walk-stop; repeat

Extending the Activity: When the children are ready, challenge them to walk in sideways and backward directions (*space*), reminding them to be even more careful when moving among their classmates. To increase the challenge, combine two movement elements, offering challenges such as the following:

- Walk forward on your heels (*space* and *shape*).
- Walk backward on tiptoe.
- Walk sideways while making your body very small.
- Walk slowly in a curving pathway (*time* and *space*).
- Walk quickly in a zigzagging pathway.
- Walk as quickly and lightly as you can (*time* and *force*).

To incorporate *rhythm*, accompany any of the above activities with "Walking Along." Don't be concerned if the children do not move "at one" with the beat of the music. It will all come in good time.

Incorporate imagery into the exploration of this locomotor skill by asking the children to walk like they are the following:

big and strong

fat and jolly like Santa Claus

really mad

really sad; tired; proud; scared

trying to find a towel with soap in
   their eyes

in a parade

on hot sand that is burning their feet

trying to get through sticky mud;
   deep snow; an overgrown jungle

Observation and Evaluation: Does the child demonstrate proper posture and alignment, with weight distributed evenly over all five toes and the heel of the foot? Does the child respond to the imagery used?

Adding Equipment: Play "Walking Along," inviting the children to accompany the song with rhythm instruments. Challenge them to roll a hoop, balance a beanbag on different body parts, or circle a ribbon stick overhead or to one side while walking.

Curriculum Connectors: By accompanying the activity with "Walking Along," you are bringing in the element of *music*. Because self-discovery, including the exploration of emotions, is the first step in *social studies* for young children, using the imagery suggested incorporates that content area. To include *language arts* and *science*, read the following poem to the children. Then ask them to act it out as you read it again. (You may have to explain and/or demonstrate what a pendulum is.)

The elephant's walk is careful and slow.
His trunk like a pendulum swings to and fro.
But when there are children with peanuts around,
He swings it up and swings it down.

Exploring Up and Down

For this initial exploration of the levels in space, pose the following questions and movement challenges:

- Do you know what "up" and "down" mean? Show me with your body.
- Show me you can make your body go all the way down. All the way up.
- How high up can you get?
- Show me you can go down halfway.
- Make yourself so tiny I can hardly see you.
- Show me you can become as huge as a giant.
- Now pretend your feet are glued to the floor. Can you move your body up and down without moving those feet?

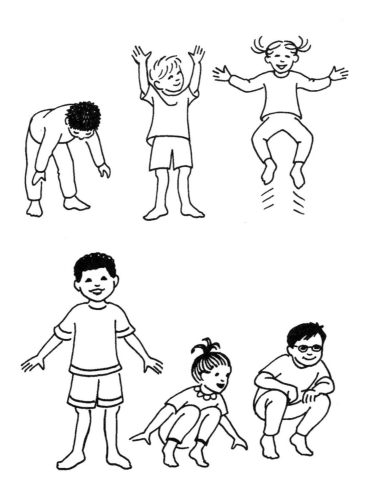

Extending the Activity: Incorporate imagery into the exploration of up and down by posing the following movement challenges:

- Pretend you are a piece of toast coming out of a toaster.
- Show me how a yo-yo moves.
- Show me you can look like a jack-in-the-box.
- Show me popcorn popping.
- Show me you can look like a bouncing ball. A seesaw. An elevator. A balloon inflating and deflating.

Any of these activities can be performed in slow motion or fast-forward (*time*). When the children are ready, invite them to move individual body parts up and down. An arm, leg, or the head are among the easiest, while parts like shoulders or elbows will be more difficult.

Observation and Evaluation: Does the child demonstrate understanding of the concepts involved? Is the child able to relate to the imagery used?

Adding Equipment: Ask the children to experiment with moving a scarf or a balloon up and down. Although this can be an introduction to the manipulative skills of throwing, catching, and volleying, you should allow the children to simply explore the possibilities at first.

Curriculum Connectors: The levels of high, low, and middle are concepts falling under the headings of both *mathematics* and *art*. Consideration of the movement in machines such as seesaws, toasters, and elevators constitutes *science*, as does experimenting with the limitations and capabilities of body parts.

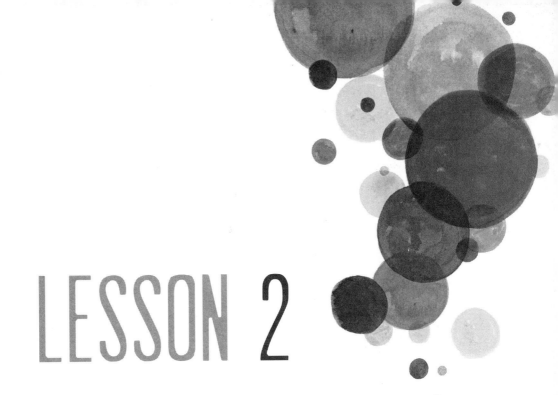

LESSON 2

Show Me

Explain to the children that this is a body-parts game like Simon Says, but you are going to say "Show me" instead—and no one will have to stop playing the game!

You can ask the children to show you a variety of body parts, including the following:

nose	knees	hips
toes	tongue	lips
eyes	tummies	shoulders
ears	hands	
elbows	chin	

Extending the Activity: Once you have addressed the list of familiar body parts, move on to more challenging parts, such as ankles, wrists, temples, thighs, and shins. You can also increase the tempo at which you call out the body parts—children love it!

Observation and Evaluation: Can the child identify body parts? Does the child demonstrate listening skills?

Adding Equipment: Provide the children with beanbags, challenging them to balance it on a variety of body parts, first while remaining in one spot and later while traveling. Beanbags can most easily be balanced on the back of the hand, a forearm, the top of the head, or a shoulder, but do not rule out the nose, elbow, and back!

Curriculum Connectors: Body-part identification is an important introductory concept for young children, falling under the theme of "My Body" and the content area of *science*, as does the concept of balance.

Let's Stretch

Have the children experiment with stretching forward, backward, toward the ceiling, and toward the floor while standing, kneeling, and sitting. Then present the following challenges and questions:

- Lie on your back and show me how long you can be.
- Can you be just as long lying on your stomach?
- Show me you can stretch wide.
- Make yourself very tiny, so tiny I can hardly see you, and then begin to "grow" very slowly, until you are as big as you can be.
- Stretch your body high while stretching your arms low.

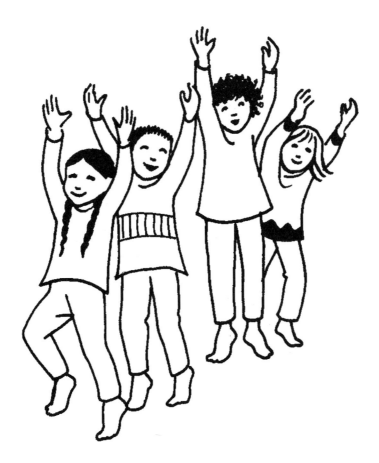

Extending the Activity: Challenge the children to discover exactly how many body parts can stretch—and in how many different directions. Remind them to stretch gently!

Observation and Evaluation: Is the child able to stretch the body parts in each of the directions presented? Does the child bend knees slightly when stretching forward at the waist?

Adding Equipment: If you have stretch bands (strips of stretchy fabric) available, invite the children to see how many different ways they can be stretched. Can they stretch them with body parts other than the hands?

Curriculum Connectors: The process of exploration and discovery is vital to *science*. You can also explore this content area further by asking the children to feel how their muscles lengthen and shorten during and after a stretch. The concept of *how many*, in the extension activity, falls under the content area of *math*.

Walking Along Again

· ·

🎵 "Walking Along Again" (Length 2:21)—CD Track 2

This song is essentially the same as "Walking Along" from Lesson 1, but it changes tempo. The children accompany the beginning of the song by walking at a normal, moderate tempo. The tempo then slows, with the children expected to also slow down. Then it is time for fast walking. Finally, the music returns to the moderate tempo.

Extending the Activity: Challenge children to modify their walk by encouraging them to walk in different shapes and pathways, and with varying amounts of force.

Developmentally, children cannot be expected to match the beat of the music at first. However, with repetitions of the activity, you can encourage them to try taking one step for every beat as they accompany the moderate tempo. When the tempo slows, they should take one step for every two beats. Finally, with the fast walking, the children will once again be taking one step per beat, but at a faster pace than at the beginning and end of the song.

Observation and Evaluation: Can the child differentiate among the moderate, slow, and fast tempos? Later, is the child able to match the beat of the music with accompanying movement?

Adding Equipment: Once children can match their movement (in this case, steps) to the music's beat, an even more challenging activity is to have them match the beat with a rhythm instrument. When children are developmentally ready, invite them to use maracas, rhythm sticks, tambourines, and hand drums as they move to this song.

Curriculum Connectors: This song explores the concepts of tempo and beat in *music*. To incorporate *social studies*, you can make this a cooperative activity. When the children are developmentally ready for the challenge, ask them to move in synchronization with a partner (for example, side by side, holding hands and matching movements).

Big and Little

Challenge children to show you the biggest and smallest shapes they can possibly make at different levels. What is the largest (smallest) shape they can make while standing? Can they find another way? What is the largest (smallest) shape(s) they can make while kneeling? Sitting? Lying down? What is the biggest (smallest) shape they can make while moving?

Extending the Activity: Read "Giants and Elves" in its entirety, explaining anything you feel needs clarification. Then divide the children into "giants" and "elves" and read the poem line by line, having the children act out their roles accordingly. If time permits, repeat the activity with the children reversing roles.

See the giants, great and tall,
Hear them bellow, hear them call.
Life looks different from up so high,
With head and shoulders clear to the sky.
And at their feet they can barely see
The little people so very tiny,
Who scurry about with hardly a care

Avoiding enormous feet placed here and
*   there.*
But together they dwell, the giants and
*   elves,*
In peace and harmony, amongst
*   themselves.*

Observation and Evaluation: Does the child demonstrate a clear difference between big and little? Is the child able to find more than one solution to each challenge? Does the child understand the concepts of shape and levels?

Curriculum Connectors: Big and little are quantitative concepts falling under the heading of *mathematics*, while the concepts of shape and levels are part of both mathematics and *art*. The poem incorporates a number of quantitative concepts and also contributes a *language arts* experience.

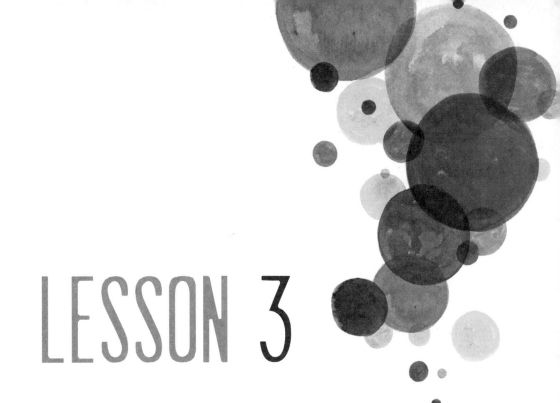

LESSON 3

My Fingers

Sit with the children and read the following poem, asking them to act out the lines as appropriate.

My Fingers

I have ten little fingers,
And they all belong to me.
I can make them do things—
Would you like to see?
I can shut them tight
Or open them wide;

I can put them together
Or make them hide.
I can make them jump high;
I can make them jump low;
I can fold them up quietly,
And hold them just so.

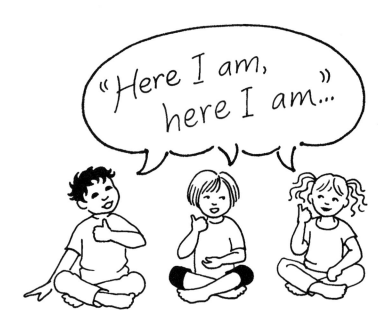

Extending the Activity: Sing "Where Is Thumbkin?" with the children, asking the whereabouts of thumbkin, pointer, middle finger, ring finger, baby finger, and the whole family, displaying the fingers appropriately.

Another option is to play a game of Counting Fingers. Ask the children to each make a fist. Then, as you count 1-2-3-4-5 very slowly, have the children open their fists to display each finger, one at a time. Then reverse, counting backward, with the children "closing" each finger one at a time. Repeat several times, counting a little faster each time.

Observation and Evaluation: Does the child demonstrate the necessary listening skills? Does the child appropriately identify fingers? Is the child able to display one finger at a time, or is more practice required?

Adding Equipment: Finger puppets can make any of these activities more fun—and colorful!

Curriculum Connectors: Poetry, of course, falls under the content area of *language arts*, as do the lyrics of "Where Is Thumbkin?" Singing the song brings in *music*, and the final activity incorporates *mathematics*. Exploring the limitations and capabilities of body parts constitutes *science*.

Bending and Stretching

Here we use imagery to explore the nonlocomotor skills of bending and stretching. Feel free to add some of your own ideas, but remember that the children must be able to relate to the images you choose.

Have the children do the following:

- Stretch as though you are picking fruit from a tall tree.
- Flop like a rag doll.
- Stretch as though you are waking up and yawning first thing in the morning.
- Bend over as though to tie shoes.
- Stretch to put something on a high shelf.
- Bend to pat a dog; an even smaller dog, or a cat.
- Stretch to shoot a basketball through a hoop.
- Bend to pick up a coin from the floor.
- Stretch as though you are climbing a ladder.
- Bend to pick vegetables or flowers from a garden.

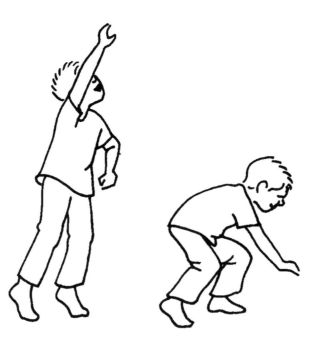

Extending the Activity: The skills are made more challenging here because the children are being asked to bend or stretch more than one body part at a time. When the children are ready, pose the following challenges:

- Stretch one arm high and the other low (one toward the ceiling and the other toward the floor).
- Bend one arm while stretching the other one high, then low, then out to the side.
- Reach both arms to the right (one side), then to the left (the other side).
- Reach one arm to the side and the other toward the ceiling.
- On your hands and knees, stretch one leg behind you and one arm forward.
- Lying on your back, stretch one leg and bend the other.
- Stretch one leg long and the other toward the ceiling.

Observation and Evaluation: Does the child differentiate between bending and stretching? Does the child identify with the imagery involved? Can the child bend and stretch in opposition, as required by the extension activities?

Curriculum Connectors: The concepts of up, down, high, and low fall under the headings of both *mathematics* and *art* (spatial relationships). Experimenting with the limitations and capabilities of body parts brings in *science*.

Let's Run

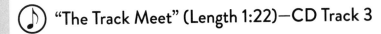

♪ "The Track Meet" (Length 1:22)—CD Track 3

Challenge the children to run in the following ways:

- in place ("Make your knees go even higher. Show me you can go faster. Now slower.")
- forward; backward
- in a circle
- making a lot of noise with the feet
- very lightly, with tiny steps
- starting and stopping on signal

Extending the Activity: Add imagery to the locomotor skill of running. Stressing realism, ask the children to run as though they are:

- carrying a football in the big game
- trying to catch a bus
- on very hot sand at the beach
- being chased by somebody
- chasing somebody
- dribbling a basketball down the court
- finishing a long, exhausting race
- flying a kite
- carrying very heavy loads on their backs

You can accompany either of these activities with "The Track Meet" to provide the children with musical motivation and an audible running rhythm. Maybe the children would like to imagine they are running in the Olympics!

Observation and Evaluation: Does the child run with the proper body alignment, with the body's weight transferred from the ball and toes of one foot to the ball and toes of the other? Is the body inclined slightly forward, with the arms bent and swinging in opposition to the legs? Does the child identify with the imagery involved?

Curriculum Connectors: Use of the song incorporates *music*, while a discussion of the Olympics can embrace *social studies*.

Bridges and Tunnels

If possible, show the children pictures of bridges and tunnels. Then ask them to show you how many ways they can form bridges and tunnels with their bodies (individually). How do bridges and tunnels differ from each other? Which is usually the rounder of the two?

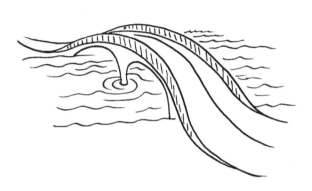 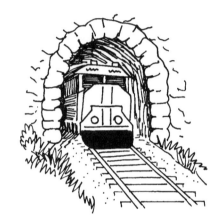

Extending the Activity: Divide the class in two, with half the children being tunnels and the other half acting as cars or trains traveling through the tunnels. Allow enough time for children to reverse roles. Another option is to sing "London Bridge" while acting it out in the traditional manner.

Observation and Evaluation: Does the child differentiate between bridges and tunnels? Does the child demonstrate both straight and round shapes? Does the child cooperate effectively with others? (*Note:* Some children may choose to show a bridge or tunnel by getting into backbends. Others with less back strength or flexibility may then try to imitate. You can discourage backbends, or backbends held too long, by inviting them to find another way to make a bridge or tunnel.)

Curriculum Connectors: Shape falls under the content areas of *mathematics* and *art*, while a discussion about transportation can bring in *social studies*. Cooperative activities also fall under the heading of social studies. Singing "London Bridge" introduces both *language arts* and *music*.

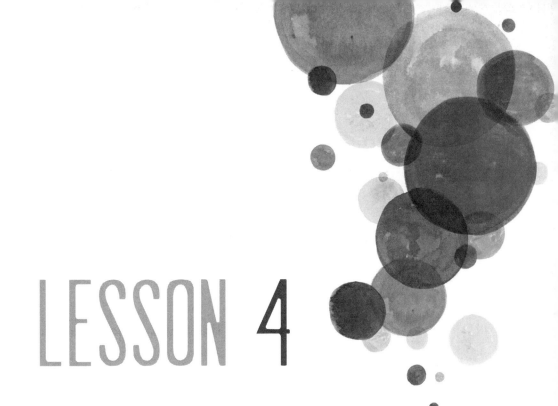

LESSON 4

See My Hands

Ask the children to sit and move their hands and fingers in the following ways:

- stretching hands and fingers as wide as possible; bending them into tightly clenched fists
- moving fingers in and out very fast; very slowly
- bringing hands together with much force (as though to clap them) but not letting them touch
- repeating the last movement, with hands up high; to one side; the other side
- bringing hands together using little force (making movement soft and light)
- clasping hands together and moving them up and down; in and out; side to side
- turning hands from front (palms) to back
- making circles with hands without moving arms

Extending the Activity: Incorporate imagery to demonstrate just how many things the hands are capable of doing and saying. Before beginning, emphasize that there is to be no touching—that they are to perform these actions "in the air." Then ask the children to show you the following things. (*Note:* Because these challenges can result in a variety of responses—divergent problem solving—you should only demonstrate yourself if the children are unable to respond.)

- praying hands
- how their hands would look if they were frightened; happy; mad
- a slapping motion
- pushing; pulling
- clapping
- calling for someone to come to them
- patting
- scolding
- fanning
- writing

- painting
- playing piano; guitar
- directing traffic
- how many ways they can wave good-bye

Observation and Evaluation: Does the child have the control necessary to perform the initial activities? Can the child accurately respond without demonstration? Does the child relate to the imagery involved?

Curriculum Connectors: Becoming familiar with the capabilities and limitations of body parts constitutes *science* for young children. Acting out feelings constitutes *social studies*.

Let's Shake

♪ "Shake It High/Shake It Low" (Length 2:58)—CD Track 4

With this exercise, children will discover they can shake various body parts, as well as the whole body, and at different levels in space. Issue the following challenges:

- Shake your whole body.
- Sit and shake just one hand; the other; both together.
- Shake your hands in front of you; to either side; up high; down low.
- Find another part of your body to shake. Then another.
- Kneeling, how many parts of your body can you find to shake?
- Lie on your back and shake one part; another; your whole body.
- Is it easier or harder to shake while lying on your tummy?

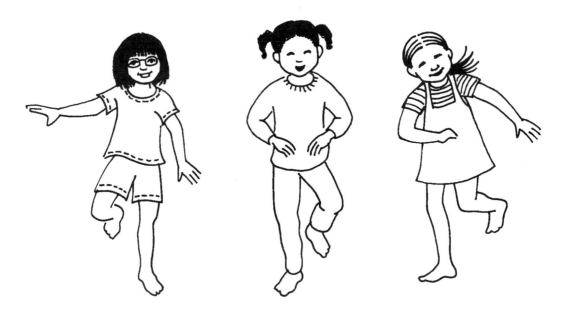

Extending the Activity: Discuss the meaning of the words *shaking*, *wiggling*, and *vibrating* with the children, and ask them to show you how they can do the following:

- move like a snake
- move like soup when the bowl is shaken
- shake and vibrate like a baby's rattle
- quiver like a leaf in the wind
- shiver as though very, very cold
- shake like a battery-powered toothbrush

"Shake It High/Shake It Low" provides some additional experience with the skill of shaking, as well as the three levels in space and the isolation of body parts. When the chorus calls for shaking "in the middle," it refers to shaking the body or part at the middle level (standing). A low level is anything lower than that, and a high level is either on tiptoe or with feet coming off the floor. Here are the lyrics:

Shaking is a way to have some fun
So let's shake our bodies, everyone!
Your head sits at the top of you;
Believe it or not, it can shake too!
There are many ways to shake a hand,
But up in the air will be just grand!
To "shake a leg" can mean to hurry
But quick or slow, no need to worry!
It can be fun to shake your bottom

So shake those hips—that's why
  you've got 'em!
Shoulders are a little bit harder,
But you can try, just for a starter!
Chorus: *Show me you can shake it high*
Show me you can shake it low
Shake it in the middle
And away we go!

Observation and Evaluation: Does the child understand the concept of shaking? Is the child able to shake a variety of body parts? Does the child relate to the imagery involved? Does the child demonstrate understanding of the three levels in space? (*Note:* Developmentally, it is still too soon to expect the children to be able to isolate individual body parts to the extent that they move *only* that part. Most likely, if a child is shaking his or her head, most of the rest of the body is also shaking!)

Adding Equipment: You might want to have maracas handy—either for demonstration purposes or to hand out to the children to add to the fun of shaking.

Curriculum Connectors: Body-part identification and experimenting with the capabilities and limitations of body parts qualifies as *science* for young children. Using the song adds both *music* and *language arts*, with exploration of the three levels in space constituting both *art* and *mathematics*.

Creepy-Crawly

· ·

Use imagery and the elements of movement to encourage the children to explore the locomotor skills of crawling (moving on the tummy) and creeping (moving on hands and knees) without their feeling "like babies." Present the following challenges, asking the children to first crawl and then creep (the movement elements being explored are cited following each set of challenges):

- Crawl (creep) forward; backward [space].
- Crawl (creep) as slowly (quickly) as you can [time].
- Crawl (creep) in a straight line [space].
- Crawl (creep) as lightly as you can [force].
- Crawl (creep) smoothly and quietly [flow and force].

Extending the Challenge: Talk to the children about the differences among the following creatures, to stimulate the most realistic responses possible. Then ask them to crawl or creep like these animals and people:

- a dog
- a cat
- a spider
- a snake
- a seal
- a baby just learning how

Observation and Evaluation: Does the child demonstrate a cross-lateral pattern (limbs used in opposition) for both crawling and creeping? Does the child differentiate between crawling and creeping?

Adding Equipment: Set up an obstacle course that includes store-bought tunnels, desks, chairs, used tires, or large, empty appliance boxes to encourage your children to get more practice with these important cross-lateral skills.

Curriculum Connectors: As mentioned in the introductory sections, cross-lateral movement has been shown to be critical to reading and writing skills (*language arts*). Moving like a variety of animals falls under the category of *science*.

Making Shapes

Shape is a movement element that is fun to explore in personal space. Making sure the children have enough room to respond without touching one another, ask them the following:

- How round can you be?
- How flat can you be? Wide? Narrow? Long? Short? Crooked? Straight?
- Can you make your body look like a table? A chair?
- Can you look like a ball? A pencil with a point at the end? A flower? A teapot? A rug?

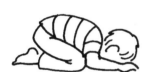 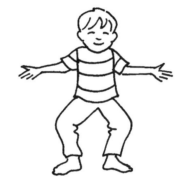 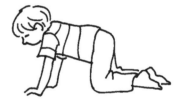

Extending the Activity: Show the children pictures of construction paper cutouts of different shapes (for example, squares, triangles, circles, rectangles), or point out items in the room (for example, a desk, a chair, the blackboard, a jacket). Then ask your preschoolers or kindergartners to imitate these shapes, one at a time, with their bodies.

Observation and Evaluation: Does the child understand the concept of shape? Is the child able to replicate shapes appropriately?

Adding Equipment: The children will have great fun trying these shapes from the insides of Body Sox (a stretchy fabric available from physical education suppliers).

Curriculum Connectors: Shape is integral to both *art* and *mathematics*. Physically replicating what the eyes are seeing, as the children are being asked to do in the alternate activity, is essential to art and writing (*language arts*).

LESSON 5

See My Face

Sit with the children and explain how they are going to discover the many different things they can do with their faces alone. Then present the following challenges to them:

- Let me see a smile; a frown.
- Make a "growling" face.
- Close your eyes real tight. Now open them wide.
- Wiggle your nose like a bunny rabbit does.
- Close your mouth real tight. Open it wide like a tunnel.
- Show me you can make your mouth move from side to side.
- Pucker up as if you have just sucked on a sour lemon.
- Blink your eyes open and shut like a light going on and off.
- Lick your lips as if you just saw something yummy to eat.
- Show me a surprised face; an angry face; a really sad, about-to-cry face; a happy face!

Extending the Activity: Play a game of Pass a Face. Sit in a circle with the children and begin by making a face that you "pass" to the child to your right or left. That child makes the *same* face and passes it along in the same direction. When the face has been passed all around the circle and comes back to you, repeat the process with a different facial expression.

You can make the activity more challenging by having each child imitate the face passed on to her or him, but then also making a *new* face, which she or he then passes on to the next child.

Observation and Evaluation: Does the child properly identify and move facial body parts? Does the child identify with the imagery used? Does the child demonstrate self-expression? Does the child physically replicate what the eyes are seeing in the activity extension?

Curriculum Connectors: Body-part identification and experiences fall under the heading of *science* for young children, while opportunities for self-expression constitute *social studies*, as does the cooperative nature of the activity extension.

Let's Sway

♪ **"The Swaying Song" (Length 2:02)—CD Track 5**

Demonstrate swaying to the children, explaining that a *sway* transfers weight from one part of the body to another in an easy, relaxed motion. Then ask them to try swaying from side to side and then back and forth.

Next, add some imagery to the activity by asking them to sway like the following things:

- flowers in the breeze
- rocking horses (or rocking chairs)
- bells ringing
- windshield wipers

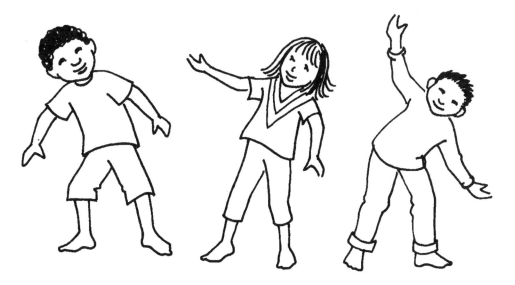

Extending the Activity: When the children are ready to perform the sway to the accompaniment of music, ask them to stand in a circle, and then put on "The Swaying Song." Ask the children to sway in the following ways:

- without touching one another
- holding hands

- with arms on one another's shoulders
- side by side with arms around one another's waists

Eventually, while the children are in the latter position, challenge them to increase the sway just a bit so one foot is coming slightly off the floor. (If they are swaying to the right, the left foot will lift, and vice versa.)

Observation and Evaluation: Does the child properly execute a sway, alone and with others? Does the child demonstrate the balance and recovery required when swaying until one foot lifts off the floor?

Adding Equipment: When moving individually, swaying a ribbon stick or streamer simultaneously can help the child correctly perform a sway by imitating the look and feel of the prop.

Curriculum Connectors: Using the song incorporates *music*. Balance and recovery are components of *science*. Swaying cooperatively qualifies as *social studies*.

Let's Jump

A jump propels the body upward from a takeoff on two feet. The toes, which are the last to leave the ground (heel-ball-toe), are the first to reach it upon landing; landings occur toe-ball-heel and with both knees bent. Ask the children to experiment with jumping in the following ways:

- in place ("Do it with your feet barely coming off the floor. With your feet coming way off. Make your knees go higher. Show me you can you jump fast. Jump being as tall as you can. As small.)
- forward ("Jump to that point over there. Jump in a circle. Now jump very slowly.")
- backward ("Make a lot of noise with your feet when you jump. Now jump very lightly, as though you are jumping on eggs and you do not want to break them.")

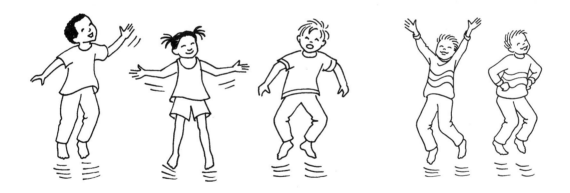

Extending the Activity: Add some imagery to the exercise, asking the children to jump in these ways:

- as though they are bouncing balls (some high, some low)
- pretending to reach for something above them
- as though they are startled by a loud noise
- as though they are angry (having a tantrum)
- with joy

A more challenging version of this activity is to invite the children to explore jumping in the following ways:

- with feet together, then apart
- with feet alternately apart and together
- landing with one foot forward and the other back
- clicking their heels together while in the air
- with arms held still by their sides
- with arms folded across the chest
- with arms extended forward, then upward, then to the sides
- with their hands on their hips
- with their hands clasped behind their backs
- with hands clapping

Observation and Evaluation: Is the child achieving elevation by pushing off from the toes? Does the child land with knees bent and heels coming all the way down to the floor? Does the child maintain a correct posture while jumping and landing?

Adding Equipment: Empty bathroom tissue rolls can be used as candlesticks to play a game of Jack (Jill) Be Nimble.

Curriculum Connectors: Incorporate *science* by discussing (in simple terms) the concept of gravity. In other words, ask the children why they do not stay up in the air when they jump. If you use the nursery rhyme "Jack Be Nimble," you will be adding a *language arts* element.

Pop Goes the Weasel

♪ "Pop Goes the Weasel" (Length 1:24)—CD Track 6

Ask children to walk to this familiar melody, jumping lightly into the air each time they hear the "pop." If you have a large enough space, you can instruct the children to walk freely about the room. Otherwise, you might suggest the group walk in a circle.

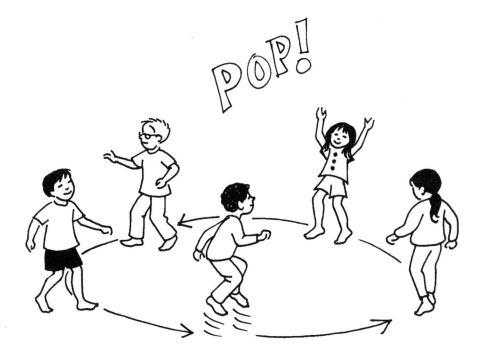

Extending the Activity: You can make this activity more challenging by asking children to change direction with each jump, to jump and clap with each pop, or to do all three at once. To fully explore the movement element of *flow*, ask the children to freeze each time they hear the pop, moving again only when the next phrase of the music begins.

Observation and Evaluation: Does the child exhibit listening skills? Does the child walk and jump with correct posture? Does the child have the self-regulation skills to stop and start on signal?

Adding Equipment: Give each of the children a hand drum or tambourine to strike on each pop.

Curriculum Connectors: These activities are primarily about listening (one of the components of *language arts*) to the *music*.

LESSON 6

...ent body-parts activity that is familiar to most children. In this activity, ... played without the elimination process. (In the traditional game, the children ...eed to participate the most are usually the first to be eliminated!) Begin by saying "Simon says" before each request.

"Simon" might make the following requests:

- Raise your arms.
- Touch your head.
- Stand up tall.
- Touch your toes.
- Touch your shoulders.
- Pucker up your mouth.
- Stand on one foot.
- Place your hands on your hips.
- Bend and touch your knees.
- Close (open) your eyes.
- Reach for the sky.
- Give yourself a hug!

Extending the Activity: To incorporate listening skills into the activity, as with the traditional game, begin saying "Simon says" only before *some* of the requests, reminding children they are not supposed to move without Simon's permission. To keep all children participating all the time, divide the group into two circles or lines. When a child moves without Simon's permission, he or she simply leaves his or her original line or circle and goes to the other one.

You can also make the game more challenging by incorporating more "difficult" body parts, like elbows, wrists, ankles, temples, and shins.

Observation and Evaluation: Can the child appropriately identify body parts? Does the child exhibit listening skills?

Curriculum Connectors: Body-part identification falls under the heading of *science* for young children, while listening skills are required in both *music* and *language arts*.

Let's Bounce

A bounce is a movement involving a rebound. Discuss this concept with the children, using the image of a ball to explain it. Then, with the children remaining in place, pose the following challenges:

- Bounce up and down like a ball.
- Bounce very lightly, barely coming off the floor.
- Bounce very hard, pushing off the floor.
- Bounce your head up and down. Do it very quickly. Now do it slowly.
- Bounce your arms up and down.

Extending the Activity: When the children are ready, challenge them to bounce such parts as elbows, fingers, and shoulders.

Adding Equipment: Demonstrating with a ball could be very helpful.

Curriculum Connectors: The concept of rebounding falls under the heading of simple *science*. Up and down are positional concepts and therefore come under the content areas of *art* and *mathematics*.

Rabbits and 'Roos

. . . .

♪ "Rabbits and 'Roos" (Length 1:44)—CD Track 7

Talk to the children about rabbits and kangaroos, discussing with them the difference in the size of these animals and, therefore, in the force of each animal's jump.

Play "Rabbits and 'Roos," having the children jump like rabbits during the "rabbit" sections of the music and like kangaroos during the "'roo" parts. The song begins with two verses for the rabbits (A) and two for the 'roos (B); the entire form is AA, BB, AA, BB, AB.

Extending the Activity: Because this activity focuses on light and heavy—and the music sets the tempo—you do not want to suggest varying the elements of force and time. However, you can suggest the children move in different directions and pathways as they pretend to be rabbits and kangaroos. Another alternative is to divide the class in two, with half acting as the rabbits and the other half as the kangaroos.

Observation and Evaluation: Is the child listening for the musical changes? Does the child demonstrate a difference between jumping lightly (like a rabbit) and jumping heavily (like a kangaroo)? Is the child executing jumps correctly?

Curriculum Connectors: In addition to *music*, this activity involves the concepts of light and heavy, which are quantitative concepts falling under the heading of *mathematics*. The focus on animals constitutes *science*.

Moving Backward

So far the children have not concentrated solely on moving in a backward direction. However, having acquired a respect for movement and for personal space, they should be ready for this activity. Reminding them to look over their shoulders, ask the children to move backward in the following ways:

- walking
- jumping
- creeping
- walking with little steps
- walking with big steps
- on hands and feet

Extending the Activity: When the children are ready, play a game of Shrinking Room, with children moving in a backward direction. With this game, you first allow the children to explore all the available space as they are moving backward, with the goal being that no one is to touch anyone else. Then, pretending you are a wall, a little bit at a time, move toward the children until they are moving in as little space as possible while still not touching one another.

Observation and Evaluation: Is the child able to move in a backward direction without bumping into anyone or anything? Does the child show respect for the personal space of others?

Adding Equipment: For Shrinking Room, you can provide each child with a plastic hoop to hold around the waist. The goal then becomes that none of the hoops will touch each other. The benefit of using hoops in this manner is that it allows children to actually *see* their own personal space, and that of others.

Curriculum Connectors: Direction is a component of *art* and *mathematics* but is also essential to reading and writing (*language arts*). The cooperative nature of Shrinking Room falls under *social studies*.

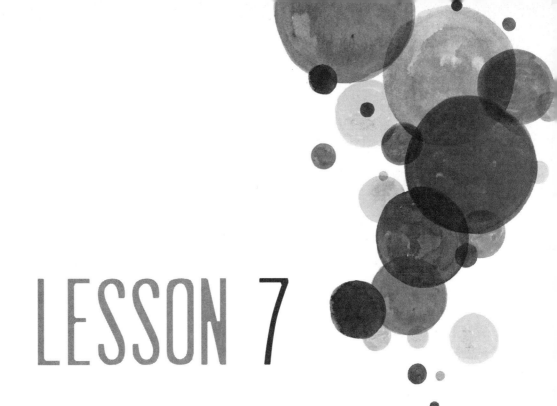

LESSON 7

The Body Song

. . . .

♪ "The Body Song" (Length 2:21)—CD Track 8

Read the following lyrics (as though they were a poem) to the children, asking them to act out the lines accordingly. To the words of the chorus, the children should run their hands down and up the length of their bodies on the first and third lines, and shrug on the second line. The fourth line is self-explanatory.

Show me you can touch your toes,	*Wiggle fingers in the air.*
Then bring your hand up to your nose.	*Shake your hips now, if you dare.*
Put a smile upon your face,	*Close your eyes, then open quick.*
Do it all in your own space.	*Around your lips let your tongue lick.*
Bring your elbows to your knees,	*With your shoulders you can shrug.*
Then shake all over, if you please.	*Give yourself a great big hug!*
Straighten up, with hands on hips.	**Chorus:** *The body, the body.*
Can you pucker up those lips?	*What parts do you know?*
Touch your ankle with your hand.	*The body, your body.*
Upon one foot can you now stand?	*Touch it high and low!*

Extending the Activity: Once the children are familiar with this activity as a poem, play "The Body Song" and do it musically. When the chorus asks, "What parts do you know?," invite children to shout out a body part, simultaneously pointing to it.

Observation and Evaluation: Can the child identify the appropriate body parts? Does the child demonstrate the necessary listening skills?

Curriculum Connectors: Body-part identification falls under the heading of *science*. This activity also involves *language arts* and *music*.

Exploring Bending and Stretching

Bending and stretching are the simplest of the nonlocomotor skills to perform, and they have already been introduced to the children. However, the skills are made more challenging here because the students are being asked to bend or stretch more than one body part at a time.

Pose the following challenges:

- Show me you can stretch one arm high and the other low (one toward the ceiling and the other toward the floor).
- Bend one arm while stretching the other arm high, then low, then out to the side.
- Reach both arms to the right (one side), then to the left (the other side).
- Reach one arm to the side and the other toward the ceiling.
- On hands and knees, stretch one leg behind you and one arm forward.
- Lying on your back, stretch one leg and bend the other.
- Stretch one leg long and the other toward the ceiling.

Extending the Activity: Invite children to discover how many other body parts can be bent and stretched—and in how many ways (reminding them to be gentle!).

Observation and Evaluation: Does the child understand the concepts of bending and stretching? Is the child able to bend and stretch in opposition? Does the child understand the directions?

Adding Equipment: Giving the children a pencil and paper to record their findings (the number of body parts they discovered can bend and/or stretch) can spark interest in the extended activity and encourage more serious probing.

Curriculum Connectors: Exploring the capabilities and limitations of body parts constitutes *science*. The concept of "how many" falls under *mathematics*. Directionality is essential to reading and writing (*language arts*).

Moving Like Animals

Talk about the characteristics of each animal listed below. Then, stressing realism, ask the children to show you how the following animals move:

- a chicken
- a monkey
- a racehorse
- a huge, heavy elephant
- a dog
- a rabbit
- a turtle
- a bird
- a lion or tiger
- a kangaroo

Extending the Activity: Read the following poem in its entirety and discuss it with the children. Then read it again, as slowly as necessary, with the children acting out the movements of each of the animals mentioned.

Let's visit a while at the local zoo,
And see what we might see.
A tall giraffe or a kangaroo,
Even a chimpanzee!
See the elephant swinging his trunk,
And hear the lion roar.
Could that black-and-white creature be
   a skunk?
Do you want to see some more?

Why, there's a gorilla in that cage.
And, my, it seems to me,
The tiger is in a terrible rage
But the bear is as calm as can be.
Well, it's getting late; but don't you fret,
We'll come back another day.
You haven't seen the hippos yet,
Or the slippery seals at play!

Observation and Evaluation: Does the child demonstrate differences in size and quality of movement (heavy versus light, speed, and so on)? Does the child show an ability to imagine?

Curriculum Connectors: The animal theme places these activities under *science*, while use of the poem incorporates *language arts*.

Moving Slow/Moving Fast

♪ "Moving Slow/Moving Fast" (Length 2:44)—CD Track 9

Play this song, consisting of slow sections (A) and fast sections (B). The form of the song is ABAB (slow, fast; slow, fast). Suggest the children move in the following ways to each tempo:

Slow Music	Fast Music
tiptoeing	fast walking
floating weightlessly	taking tiny steps
taking soft, giant steps	shaking all over
swaying	jumping lightly

Extending the Activity: Once children can easily recognize the difference in tempo, encourage them to find their own ways of moving to the slow and fast music. Does the music make them feel like moving in different ways?

When children are familiar with the contrast between fast and slow, ask them to pretend to be things that are either fast or slow. You may choose to complete one category before moving to the other, or you can alternate between the two categories. Generally, young children will find it easier to perform fast movements.

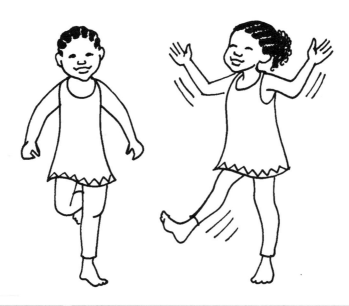

Fast	Slow
a fire engine	a turtle
a jet plane	the hands of a clock
an arrow	a snail
the wind	a train just starting up
a cheetah	the sun rising
a spaceship	a snowman melting

Observation and Evaluation: Can the child recognize the difference between the slow and fast tempos? Do the child's movements show a marked difference between slow and fast? Does the child identify with the imagery used?

Adding Equipment: Giving children a prop to move, such as a scarf, streamer, or ribbon stick, can help alleviate any self-consciousness and also allows them to see the difference between slow and fast movements.

Curriculum Connectors: This song explores the concept of tempo in *music* and the movement element of time, which falls under the heading of *mathematics* for young children. The self-expression involved adds a touch of *social studies*.

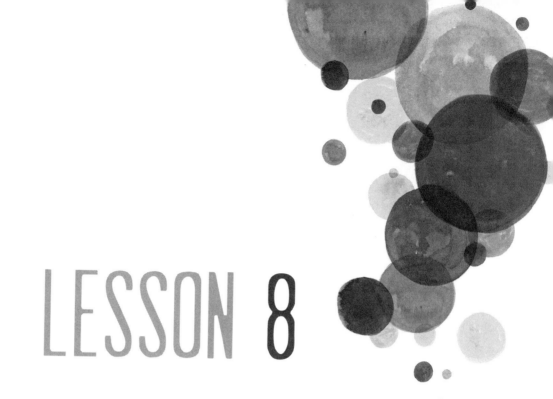

LESSON 8

Mirror Game

As part of their development, children must learn to imitate physically what they experience visually. This game gives them the opportunity to do just that.

Standing where all of the children can easily see you, explain that they should pretend to be your reflection in the mirror, imitating your every move. You then move parts of your body in various ways (for example, raising and lowering an arm, tilting your head) slowly and without verbal instruction; and the children do likewise.

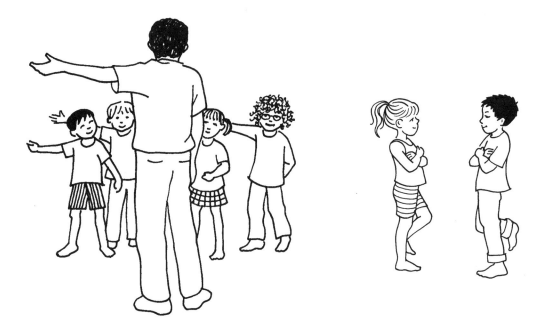

Extending the Activity: When the children are ready to work in partners, ask them to pair off and stand facing each other. One child performs a series of simple movements (standing in place), which the second child mirrors. After a while, partners reverse roles.

Observation and Evaluation: Is the child able to imitate what her or his eyes are seeing? Does the child cooperate effectively with a partner?

Curriculum Connectors: Being able to replicate physically what the eyes are seeing is a central component of *art* and writing (*language arts*). The cooperative nature of the extended activity brings it into *social studies*.

Let's Turn

Children love to turn themselves around and even to make themselves dizzy. In this activity, however, they will be introduced to the nonlocomotor skill of turning as a *controlled* movement—a rotation of the body around an axis that can occur in a great variety of ways.

Pose the following questions and challenges:

- Turn yourself around to the right (one way). Now turn to the left (the other way).
- Turn yourself around very, very slowly.
- Turn while making yourself as tall (small) as you can.
- Show me you can you turn while you are on your knees. On one knee.
- Turn while sitting on your bottom.
- Turn on just one foot.
- Can you jump and turn at the same time?

Extending the Activity: Additional challenges include the following:

- Turn the way an airplane would as it comes in for a landing.
- Hop and turn at the same time.
- Turn while on one knee.
- Turn while making yourself as round (crooked) as you can be.
- Turn quickly, and then very gradually slow down.

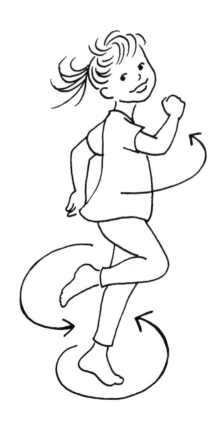

Observation and Evaluation: A turn is a partial or complete rotation of the body around an axis, causing a shift in weight placement. Does the child display an ability to correctly execute half and full turns with control and in a variety of ways?

Adding Equipment: Executing turns while standing inside a hoop can help children understand that turning is a nonlocomotor skill. It is also fun to turn while holding a streamer or ribbon stick.

Curriculum Connectors: The concept of rotation around an axis is simple *science*, as is the balance involved in these activities.

Marching Band

 "Marching Band" (Length 2:55)—CD Track 10

Play this song and ask the children to march in the following ways. Don't be concerned if they do not step in time with the beat—it's early yet!

- in place, raising their knees high
- in place, turning in one direction, then turning in the other direction
- as though they are playing an imaginary instrument
- as though they are carrying a flag in a parade

Extending the Activity: When the children are ready, challenge them to march around the room to the song. Possible challenges include marching in the following ways:

- with knees high and arms swinging
- as though in a parade
- as though playing an instrument in a parade
- in a square path around the room (changing direction at every corner)

Observation and Evaluation: Does the child have a sense of the 1-2 rhythm of marching? Does the child maintain correct posture while marching?

Adding Equipment: Marching and playing an instrument at the same time is more developmentally challenging than doing either alone, but children love the opportunity to play a rhythm instrument.

Curriculum Connectors: A march is a style of *music*. Any discussion of the holidays during which parades are held can bring in *social studies*. Directionality is a critical component of reading and writing (*language arts*), and the square pattern in the extension activity adds a touch of *math*.

Exploring Body and Spatial Directions

Ask the children to each find their own personal space and to remember where that space is. Then stand in the center of the room where everyone can see you, acting as a point of reference, and present the following challenges:

- Walk to me, turn, and go back to your own space.
- Walk forward to me, but return to your space sideways.
- Walk sideways to me and return to your space backward.
- Walk backward to me and return to your space in a forward direction.

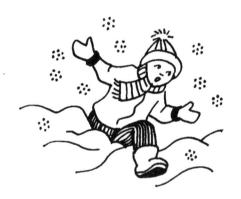 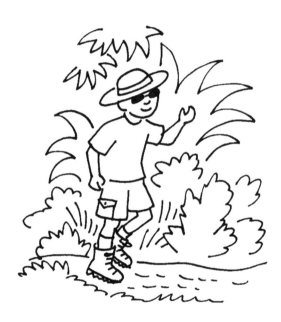

Extending the Activity: You can further challenge children to approach and retreat from you in the following ways:

- in a straight path
- from one side, then from the other side
- from the back
- in a curving path, then in a zigzagging one

Ask the children to really use their imaginations by challenging them to approach and retreat from you as though they are in the following situations:

- on slippery ice
- on hot sand that is burning their feet
- in deep snow
- in sticky mud
- on the moon and weightless
- in a jungle with thick growth
- on a busy, crowded sidewalk

Observation and Evaluation: Does the child demonstrate the ability to move in the directions cited? Can the child move without interfering with the movement of others? Does the child identify with the imagery used?

Adding Equipment: Using hoops, carpet squares, or poly spots (available from movement education suppliers) can help children identify and remember their own personal spaces.

Curriculum Connectors: Direction and space are components of *art*, and a sense of direction aids reading and writing (*language arts*). The self-expression required in the extension activity brings in *social studies*.

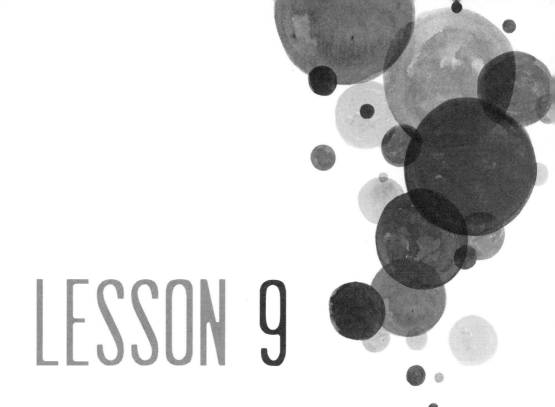

LESSON 9

Hands-Hands-Hands

· ·

♪ "Hands-Hands-Hands" (Length 2:46)—CD Track 11

Read the following poem to the children, having them act out the lines accordingly. You may also want to emphasize the fact that these movements are to be performed without touching another person.

Would you like to have some fun with your
   hands?
There are many things they can do.
They can push and pull and lead a band,
And that's just to name a few!
They can make fists that shake in the air
When you're mad as you can be.
They reach out to show someone you care
By touching him tenderly.
A hand is something that bounces a ball
And it turns the page of a book.

It dials the phone when you make a call
And puts it back on the hook.
With your hand you pet your favorite cat
And feel the softness of fur.
It's your hands that hold your baseball bat
And with a spoon help you stir.
Can you show me a drummer when she plays
Or somebody scrubbing pans?
Can you think of a few other ways
That you just might use your hands?

(*Note:* The lyrics of the song talk about dialing a phone and putting it back on the hook. You may need to explain about older phones.)

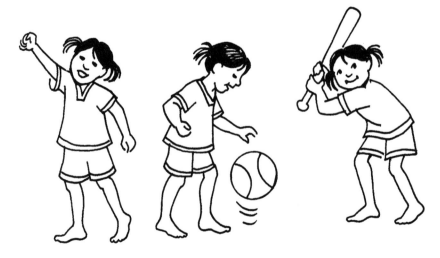

Extending the Activity: When the children are ready to perform this activity musically, familiarize them with the chorus, instructing them to open and close their hands three times during its first and third lines.

The chorus is as follows:

Hands-hands-hands
They shake and scold and pat.
Hands-hands-hands
They wave and pray and clap.

Observation and Evaluation: Does the child respond appropriately to the images used? Does the child exhibit the necessary listening skills? Is the child able to keep up when the activity is performed musically?

Curriculum Connectors: These activities offer experiences in *music, language arts* (listening and word comprehension), and self-expression, which comes under the heading of *social studies.*

Let's Sit

Although sitting may be a skill preschoolers and kindergartners have long since mastered, it can still be a challenging activity when explored at a variety of levels, especially if you incorporate the additional movement elements of time and force. Explain this to the children, and then present the following challenges:

- Sit from a standing position, using your hands to let you down.
- Do it again, this time without using your hands.
- Sit down very slowly.
- Sit with a thump.
- Sit with the weight on your right (left) thigh.

Extending the Activity: Additional challenges might include the following:

- Sit—gently—from a kneeling position.
- Again from a kneeling position, sit down with a thump.
- From a kneeling position, sit with the weight on your right (left) thigh.
- Sit up from a lying position.
- Show me how slowly you can sit up from a lying position.

Observation and Evaluation: Does the child demonstrate the control necessary to perform these tasks? Does the child understand what is expected?

Adding Equipment: Performing these tasks within a hoop or on a poly spot can make them more visual and colorful, thereby making them more fun.

Curriculum Connectors: These activities move the children through the levels in space, which qualifies them as *mathematics* experiences. Act out the nursery rhyme "Little Miss (Mister) Muffet," with children acting as the lead character and/or the spider, to incorporate *language arts*.

Let's Leap

A leap is similar to a run, except that the knee and ankle action is greater to create spring. Preschoolers and kindergartners may be able to relate best to this locomotor skill through imagery. For example, you can ask them to pretend to leap in the following ways:

- over a puddle
- over a tall building (like a superhero)
- like a deer over fallen trees in the forest
- as though leaping over a hurdle in the Olympics

Extending the Activity: Children will first lead with the preferred (easier) leg. Be sure to encourage them to try leaping with the nonpreferred (more difficult) leg leading as well.

After the children have had ample experience with leaping, challenge them to combine leaping with running. Ask them to do these movements:

- perform several leaps in a row without stops in between
- run several steps, and then leap; repeat
- run, leap; run, leap; and so on
- run, run, leap; run, run, leap; and so on

Observation and Evaluation: Does the child differentiate between leaping and jumping? Following takeoff, does the child lead with the knee and then extend it as the foot reaches forward to land? Does the back leg extend to the rear while the child is in the air? Does the child raise the arms to assist with elevation?

Adding Equipment: Some children relate better to leaping when it is performed over a prop, like a rope held just an inch or two off the floor. Again, be sure they practice leading with both legs.

Curriculum Connectors: Discuss the concept of gravity with the children, reminding them that it is the reason they do not stay in the air when they leap, to bring in *science*. The concept of "over" is both a positional one (*mathematics*) and a preposition (*language arts*).

Moving Softly/Moving Loudly

♪ "Moving Softly/Moving Loudly" (Length 2:47)—CD Track 12

The form of this song is ABAB, with A being the soft section. Offer the following suggestions to the children, one at a time, as they move to the music:

Soft	Loud
tiptoeing	stamping feet
moving arms gently	punching toward the
patting the floor	sky
swaying gently	pounding the floor
	rocking forcefully

Extending the Activity: Once children can distinguish between soft and loud music, challenge them to move any way they like to the soft and loud sections. Can they find new ways to move?

Observation and Evaluation: Can the child distinguish between soft and loud? Does the child demonstrate movements appropriate to soft and loud music?

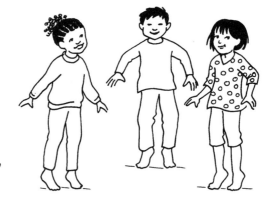

Adding Equipment: How might a prop, such as a scarf, streamer, or ribbon stick, move to the soft and loud music?

Curriculum Connectors: This activity involves the concept of volume (*music*) and the movement element of force, which is a concept falling under both *mathematics* and *science*. Listening is one of the four components of *language arts*.

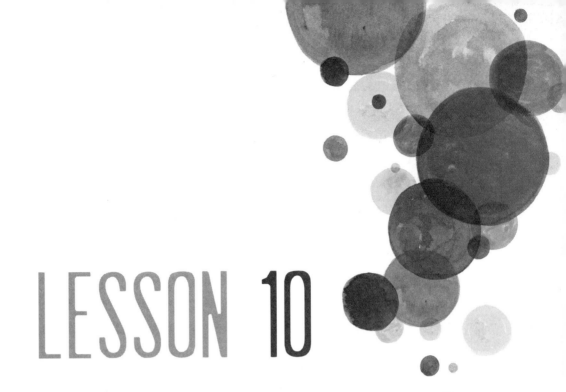

LESSON 10

A Face Has Many Roles in Life

. . . .

♪ **"A Face Has Many Roles in Life" (Length 3:19)—CD Track 13**

This poem requires the children to express themselves with only their faces. Read it aloud, asking them to show you the emotions cited.

A face has many roles in life,
I guess you know that's true.
It smiles and frowns and even cries
When you are feeling blue.
A face can show that you're angry;
A face can show you're glad.
A face can pout and sulk and whine
When you are feeling bad.

A face can show that you're tired
With yawns or drooping eyes.
A face can even show delight
When someone yells, "Surprise!"
A face has many roles in life,
But most unique by far—
'Cause yours belongs to only you
I can tell who you are!

Extending the Activity: When the children are ready, do the activity as a song, first familiarizing them with the chorus. During it, have them point to (or move) the parts named. On the next-to-last line, they can cover their faces with their hands, then uncover them on the last line to display an expression or funny face of their choice.

The chorus is:

A nose, a mouth, a couple of eyes,
Two eyebrows that you raise.
These belong to any face,
But you use them in your own ways!

Observation and Evaluation: Does the child demonstrate an ability for self-expression?

Curriculum Connectors: These activities offer experiences with *language arts*, *music*, and self-expression, which falls under the content area of *social studies* for young children.

Let's Push and Pull

Discuss pushing and pulling with the children, particularly the aspect of *resistance* that is part of both of these skills. With this activity, the children will be pretending to push and pull a number of objects of differing weights and sizes. Emphasizing that these exercises are imaginary and must be performed without the children touching one another, ask them to move as though they are doing the following:

- pushing a swing
- pulling a rope
- pushing heavy furniture
- pulling a kite
- pushing a balloon into the air
- pulling an anchor out of the water
- pushing a car stuck in mud or snow
- pulling a wagon or sled
- pushing a lawn mower
- pulling in a game of tug-of-war
- pushing a shovel
- pulling a balloon down from the sky
- pushing a grocery cart

Extending the Activity: The following challenges should be presented twice—once for pushing and then again for pulling, so the children have a chance to experience the contrast. Ask them to push (pull) in these ways:

- with both hands
- with one hand and then the other, alternately
- forward, downward, upward, sideways
- strong and hard; then lightly (against less resistance)
- very slowly; then quickly
- with short (long) movements

Observation and Evaluation: Does the child identify with the imagery used? Does the child differentiate between pushing and pulling? Does the child understand the concept of resistance and demonstrate the proper amount of muscle tension?

Curriculum Connectors: The concept of resistance is relative to *science*.

Let's Gallop

 "Giddy-Up" (Length 1:39)—CD Track 14

A gallop is a locomotor skill that differs from the walk and the run in that it is performed with an uneven rhythm. It is a combination of a walk and a leap in which one foot leads and the other plays catch-up.

Introduce the children to the gallop, keeping in mind that it is best learned by imitation or by holding hands and moving with someone who knows how to gallop. For those children who are not ready to perform an actual gallop, you can simply suggest moving "like a horse."

Extending the Activity: Play the song "Giddy-Up" and have the children "saddle up and ride." If space is a problem, you may want to have them gallop in a circle or in rounds, one small group at a time. The song offers brief rest periods to prepare the next group to begin or for "stopping at a watering hole."

Once children have mastered leading with the preferred foot, challenge them to lead with the other foot.

Observation and Evaluation: Does the child consistently lead with one foot, with the other following (but not passing)? Is the child's galloping rhythm uneven? Can the child lead with the nonpreferred foot?

Adding Equipment: Old-fashioned stick horses always contribute to the fun of galloping!

Curriculum Connectors: A discussion of how horses move can bring a bit of *science* to this activity, which also offers experience with *music*. Rhythm is an important element not only in music but also in *language arts*.

Marching Slow/Marching Fast

♪ **"Marching Slow/Marching Fast" (Length 2:24)—CD Track 15**

The children have had previous experience with marching to "Marching Band" (page 89). "Marching Slow/Marching Fast," however, offers two different marching tempos, requiring more bodily control—and greater listening skills—from the children.

For this lesson, simply play the song and march with the children accordingly. The form of the song is ABAB, with A being the slow march and B the fast march.

Extending the Activity: Once children can distinguish between the slow and fast tempos, invite them to march on their own, matching their tempo to that of the music. When they are demonstrating success, encourage them to try different pathways and directions.

Observation and Evaluation: Does the child distinguish between slow and fast? Do the child's movements match the music's tempo? Does the child maintain proper posture while marching?

Adding Equipment: Again, adding rhythm instruments to the mix can make the activity even more fun.

Curriculum Connectors: In addition to experiences with *music* and the movement element of time (*mathematics*), you can incorporate *social studies* by holding a discussion about those holidays that are typically celebrated with parades.

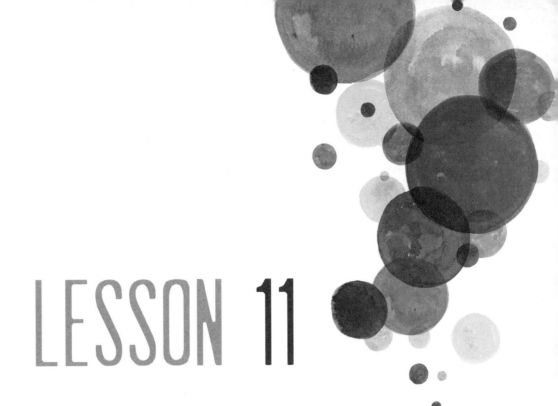

LESSON 11

Switcheroo!

This body-parts activity is played in pairs, with partners standing back to back. When you call out the name of a body part (or parts), the children turn to face each other, briefly connect those parts, and then return to their back-to-back position. When you call out "Switcheroo!" children must get back to back with a new partner, and the game begins again as you call out more body parts.

Possible "connections" to be made include the following:

- hands (both, right, or left)
- knees
- elbows
- feet
- wrists
- right or left hips
- right or left ankles
- big toes
- pointer (ring, baby) fingers

Extending the Activity: This game can be made more challenging by playing it in trios. You can also challenge the children to connect nonmatching parts (for example, a hand to a knee).

Observation and Evaluation: Does the child properly identify body parts? Does the child work cooperatively with others? Is the child ready to identify right from left?

Curriculum Connectors: Body-part identification falls under the heading of *science*, while the cooperative aspect constitutes *social studies*.

Let's Strike

A strike is a strong movement of the arm (or arms) propelled in any direction for the purpose of hitting an object. The arm must bend to initiate the strike, extending with both force and speed.

Before exploring this skill, discuss "pretending" with the children, emphasizing that their strikes are to take place *in the air* only! Then ask them to strike as though doing the following:

- playing a big bass drum in a marching band
- hammering a nail
- chopping wood
- feeling angry
- swatting at a mosquito
- hitting a ball with a bat

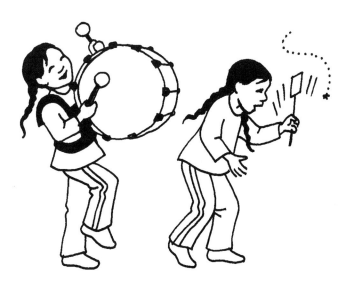 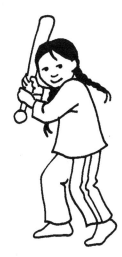

Extending the Activity: Challenge the children to strike in the following ways, while standing, kneeling, and sitting:

- with both arms
- with one (the other) arm
- alternating arms
- upward; downward; sideways
- with long (short; medium) extension of the arms

Observation and Evaluation: Does the child demonstrate the force and speed required to correctly execute a strike? Does the child identify with the imagery used? Is the child able to perform a strike in all directions and with both arms?

Adding Equipment: Because hand-eye coordination is not fully developed until age nine or ten, preschoolers and kindergartners will require much practice before being able to successfully strike an object with an implement. You can offer them opportunities to first practice striking with the hands alone (known as volleying) by providing medium to large balloons, which are lightweight and colorful (helpful for visual tracking). Challenge children to hit the balloons upward and forward with both hands. The next step is to volley the balloon with just one (the preferred) hand, then try it with the nonpreferred hand. Finally, provide each child with a short-handled paddle with which to strike the balloon.

Curriculum Connectors: *Mathematics* experiences are included with directions and such quantitative concepts as long and short. To incorporate *science*, ask the children to consider the amount of muscle tension involved in striking properly. Challenge them to experiment to see what happens when they use much less muscle tension. To incorporate *social studies*, invite the children to take partners and volley a balloon back and forth, emphasizing the cooperative nature of the activity.

Follow the Leader

Follow the Leader is performed here in the usual manner, giving the children a chance once again to observe movement and imitate what they are seeing.

The first time this activity is performed, you should act as the leader, using a variety of locomotor skills (walking, running, jumping, galloping) and pathways (straight, curving, and zigzagging). Emphasize that the children are to imitate what you are doing as closely as possible.

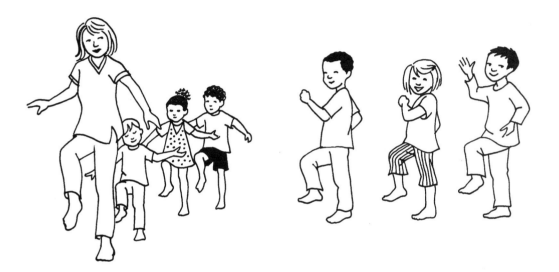

Extending the Activity: As the children acquire the ability to perform more locomotor skills, repeat this game, incorporating the new movements into it. Also continue to vary the ways in which the movements are performed (for example, lightly, heavily, quickly, slowly, and so on).

Once the children are ready for the responsibility of being line leaders, play a game of Calling Names. The children once again form a line behind you, and you begin to lead. After a while you call out the name of one of the children, and he or she breaks away from the line, followed by those behind him or her. This second line begins making its own path around the room. Continue in this manner, with each new group following its own path and being careful not to intersect another line. It is less confusing if you call the names of children toward the end of the line at first, those who have only a few other children behind them.

Observation and Evaluation: Is the child able to physically replicate what the eyes are seeing? In what way(s) is the child unable to respond? (In other words, what movement skills and/or elements require additional attention?)

Adding Equipment: To make the activity more challenging, you can include *prop* movement, which the children must also replicate. Possible props are scarves, ribbon sticks, or rhythm band instruments.

Curriculum Connectors: Being able to physically replicate what the eyes see is central to writing (*language arts*) and *art*. Language arts are also involved as children explore such adverbs as lightly, slowly, and so forth. Using rhythm band instruments will offer experience with elements of *music*.

High and Low

 "High and Low" (Length 1:50)—CD Track 16

Have the children sit on the floor. Play a bit of this song for the children. Ask them to listen for the sound that gets higher and lower. Once they can identify it, return to the beginning of the song. As the music gradually gets higher and higher, the children should raise their arms. Then they lower their arms with the descending music and rest them where the song provides for it. The pattern follows. If it seems complicated, don't worry; the rising and falling of the music is obvious.

8 counts up; 8 counts down
8 counts up; 8 counts down
8-count rest

4 counts up; 4 counts down
4 counts up; 4 counts down
8-count rest

2 counts up; 2 counts down; repeat twice
8-count rest

8 counts up; 4 counts down
4 counts up; 4 counts down
8-count rest

2 counts up; 8 counts down; repeat
2 counts up

Extending the Activity: When the children are ready, ask them to crouch low to the ground as you start the song. As the music gradually gets higher and higher, so do the children. They then descend with the music and rest where the song provides for it. Do this with the children at first, then challenge them to do it with the music only as their guide.

Observation and Evaluation: Can the child hear the rising and descending pitch? Does the child respond appropriately?

Adding Equipment: When the children are first doing this song with arms alone, you can make the activity a more "colorful" experience by providing them with two scarves apiece—one per hand. Later you could add a parachute to the whole-body experience. During the 8-count rests, instead of merely waiting, the children can circle the parachute, using whatever traveling skill they prefer (for example, walking, sliding, skipping).

Curriculum Connectors: These activities deal mainly with the concept of pitch in *music* and with the levels in space, which fall under the heading of *art*. High and low are also quantitative concepts in *mathematics*, and active listening is one of the four components of *language arts*.

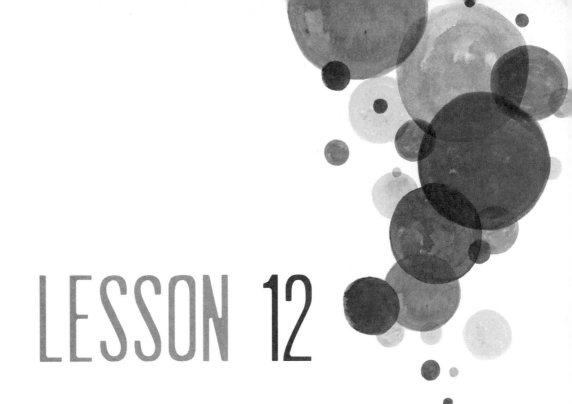

LESSON 12

Body-Part Relationships

In this activity, the children are going to work with a variety of body parts in relation to other body parts or to the floor. This will require them to think a bit more about the sum of their parts and about the space they occupy.

Ask the children to sit, and then present the following challenges:

- Put an elbow on the floor; take it as far away from the floor as possible.
- Stretch a foot far away from you, and then bring it back without touching the floor (until it is back in its original position).
- Put a shoulder (the other shoulder; both shoulders) on the floor.
- Touch an elbow to a knee; take it as far away from that knee as possible.
- Touch an elbow to a foot.
- Can you touch your foot to your shoulder?
- Touch a wrist to an ankle.

Extending the Activity: Additional challenges could include the following:

- Come up from the floor with your head leading and the rest of your body following.
- Go back down with an elbow leading the way.
- Come up from the floor with an elbow leading.
- Go back down to the floor with your nose leading the way.
- Come back up with a nose leading.
- Go back down with your chest leading.
- Come back up with your chin leading.

Observation and Evaluation: Does the child have the body and spatial awareness necessary to successfully complete these challenges? Does the child properly identify body parts?

Curriculum Connectors: This body-part experimentation falls under the heading of *science* for young children. Because it also explores personal space and levels, it involves *art* and *mathematics* concepts as well.

Let's Lift

A lift transports an object from one place to another, often from a lower to a higher level. Remind the children that they must bend their knees, straightening their legs as they lift from low to high. Then explain that they are going to pretend to lift imaginary objects of varying sizes, weights, and so on.

Ask the children to show you what it would look like to lift the following things:

- a big heavy rock
- a big beach ball
- a chair
- a log
- a basket
- a balloon
- the handles of a wheelbarrow
- something very hot

Extending the Activity: Ask the children to pretend to lift something in these ways:

- with both hands, with one hand, then with the other
- from low to high, then high to low
- from front to back, then back to front
- very slowly, then more quickly
- with great effort, then with little effort

Observation and Evaluation: Does the child bend the knees, straightening them with the lift? Does the child differentiate among the imaginary items to be lifted and respond appropriately?

Adding Equipment: If you feel that lifting imaginary objects is too abstract for your children, you can begin by providing a variety of actual items of differing shapes and sizes that they can use to practice lifting. Instruct them to pay attention to the amount of muscle tension required with each lift. Possible objects include a beach ball, pail, small chair, balloon, and a very short (light) stack of books.

Curriculum Connectors: Challenging children to focus on the muscle tension involved with these lifts constitutes *science*. The positional concepts fall under the heading of early geometry (*mathematics*), and the self-expression required qualifies as *social studies*.

Shadow Game

· ·

This is a partner activity similar to the Mirror Game played in pairs. With this game, one child stands with her or his back to the second child and performs various movements that the latter mimics, as a "shadow." Then they trade roles. These movements should all be performed with the children remaining in one place. You might want to talk to the children about shadows before beginning this activity.

Extending the Activity: When the children are ready, invite them to perform the activity while moving around the room as person and shadow. Again, they should switch roles.

Observation and Evaluation: Is the child able to physically replicate what the eyes are seeing? Does the child work cooperatively with a partner?

Curriculum Connectors: The cooperative nature of these activities place them under *social studies*, while the concept of shadows belongs to *science*. Also, the ability to physically replicate what the eyes see is central to *art* and writing (*language arts*).

Robots and Astronauts

. . . .

♪ **"Robots and Astronauts" (Length 3:19)—CD Track 17**

Play this song, the form of which is ABAB. During A, the children pretend to move like robots (stiffly and mechanically). During B, they pretend to float in space like weightless astronauts.

Extending the Activity: With repetitions of this activity, you can make it a bit more challenging by issuing follow-up questions to vary the children's responses. For example, you might ask the following:

- Is there some way those robots might use their heads as they move?
- Is there another direction (pathway) the robots might move in?
- Can the astronauts float in different directions?
- Is there another shape the astronauts might float in?

Observation and Evaluation: This is an exercise in both flow (bound and free) and force. Does the child differentiate between the bound movement of the robot and the free movement of the astronaut? Does the child exhibit a difference in muscle tension from one to the other?

Curriculum Connectors: This song explores the concept of form as well as the contrast between *staccato* (short, separated notes) and *legato* (smooth-flowing notes) in *music*. Focusing on muscle tension offers an experience in *science*. The self-expression the children display falls under the content area of *social studies*.

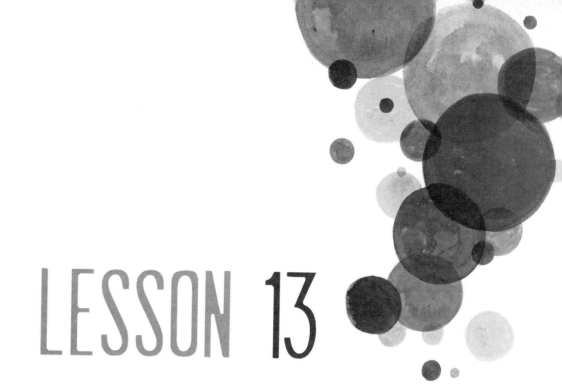

LESSON 13

Traveling Body Parts

This activity will give your preschoolers or kindergartners a better idea of the range of their personal space. Ask them to perform the following tasks while standing:

- Make one hand travel far away from the other one.
- Leaving the first hand (the one that traveled) where it is, bring the other hand to meet it.
- Make the first hand travel far away from the other one but in a different direction.
- Make one elbow travel far away from the other one.
- Leaving the first elbow where it is, bring the other elbow to meet it.
- Make the first elbow travel far away again, but in a different direction.

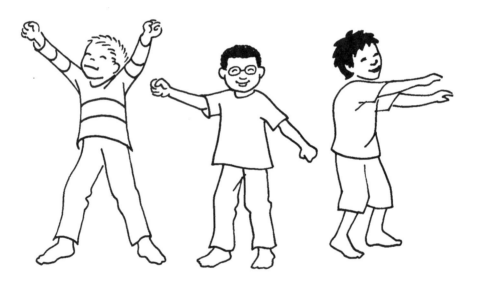

Extending the Activity: Have the children sit and repeat the preceding sequence with knees and feet.

Observation and Evaluation: Does the child understand the concepts of *apart* and *together*, *far* and *near*? Does the child have the bodily control necessary to successfully complete these tasks?

Adding Equipment: For the initial activity, holding a scarf or rhythm stick in each hand may make this activity less abstract for some children.

Curriculum Connectors: Together, apart, far, and near are important positional concepts in both *mathematics* and *art*. Experimenting with the capabilities and limitations of body parts qualifies as *science*.

Let's Swing

Swinging is one of the six qualities of movement, and it takes the form of an arc or a circle around a stationary base. A swing generally requires impulse and momentum, except perhaps when the swinging part is merely released to the force of gravity. Swinging movement can be executed by the body as a whole, by the upper or lower torso alone, and by the head, arms, or legs.

Introduce the children to swinging motion by presenting the following challenges:

- Swing your arms back and forth.
- Show me you can swing them more slowly. More quickly.
- Swing them from side to side.
- Swing your head from side to side, as though it were a windshield wiper.
- Swing your body like "the man [or woman] on the flying trapeze."
- Swing your arms like an elephant's trunk.

Extending the Activity: Have each child hold on to something (a desk or the wall) with one hand and experiment with swinging the outside leg in the following ways:

- with little (great big) swings
- slowly, then quickly
- very forcefully, then very lightly

This activity isolates the arms from the rest of the body while giving the children further opportunity to practice swinging. Begin by asking them to stand and let their arms hang loosely and heavily from their shoulders. Then issue the following challenges:

- With your arms still hanging, let them swing back and forth in a small arc (a little).
- Show me you can swing them a little more.
- Swing your arms from side to side.
- Bend forward a little, letting your arms hang down. Show me you can swing them forward and backward.
- Swing them from side to side, starting with a small arc and gradually increasing its size.

Observation and Evaluation: Does the child demonstrate the impulse and momentum required to successfully perform a swing? Can the child execute a swing with all parts of the body capable of swinging?

Adding Equipment: Providing each child with a ribbon stick or streamer can help children see the shape of an arc when the arms are swinging.

Curriculum Connectors: Experimenting with the capabilities and limitations of body parts qualifies as *science*, as does discussing and demonstrating pendulums.

Locomotion I

♪ "Locomotion I" (Length 3:28)—CD Track 18

This song asks children to pretend to move from place to place by imagining various modes of transportation. The lyrics are as follows:

Hey, everybody—look at me
And see what I can do.
I can drive a car like Dad's
And drive it carefully too!
Hey, everybody—look at me
And see what I can do.
I can ride upon a horse
And gallop lightly too!
Hey, everybody—look at me
And see what I can do.
I can engineer a train
And blow the whistle too!

Hey, everybody—look at me
And see what I can do.
I can surf on little waves
And surf on big ones too!
Hey, everybody—look at me
And see what I can do.
I can fly a big jet plane
And land it gently too!
Hey, everybody—look at me
And see what I can do.
I can lie in a big sailboat
And wave good-bye to you!

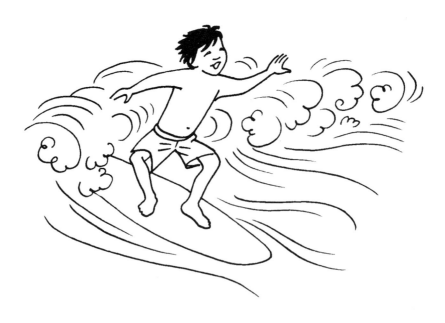

Extending the Activity: Invite the children to demonstrate other modes of transportation. To make problem solving part of the activity, ask them to depict modes of transportation found only in cities, in the air, or on the water.

Observation and Evaluation: Does the child identify with the imagery used? Does the child respond appropriately through movement?

Curriculum Connectors: In addition to *music* and *language arts*, this song, because of its focus on transportation, also offers a *social studies* experience.

Exploring Force

The element of force concerns how heavily or lightly a movement is performed and the muscle tension involved in each. The following activities will familiarize the children with this element.

Ask the children to do the following:

- Move very softly like a feather floating.
- Move very strongly, making lots of noise with your feet.
- Make strong movements with your arms like propellers on a helicopter.
- Make light arm movements like the wings of a bird sailing gently through the sky.
- Show me how hard you can push against the floor.
- Tighten up all your muscles; now move stiffly like a robot.
- Be a floppy rag doll, with no muscles holding up your body.

Extending the Activity: A wonderful relaxation exercise to get children to contract and release their muscles alternately is to have them depict a statue and then a rag doll. Always end with the rag doll!

Observation and Evaluation: Is there a clear difference between the child's strong and light movement? Does the child understand the concept of greater or lesser muscle tension for strong and light movement?

Curriculum Connectors: Light and heavy are quantitative concepts falling under the heading of *mathematics* for young children. The exploration of muscle tension constitutes *science*.

LESSON 14

ing Right and Left

. . . .

n this lesson the children are simply going to be introduced to *laterality* (preference or dominance of using the left or right side of the body) by experimenting with movements performed on one side of the body that are imitated on the other side. You should stand facing the children, pointing out to them when they are working with their right and left sides, and using your opposite side to act as a mirror reflection.

Suggest the following movements (remembering to repeat them on both sides):

- Raise and lower an arm.
- Move your arm in a smooth, wavy way.
- Lift your leg forward, and then put it back on the floor.
- Lift your leg to the side and put it back.
- Wiggle the fingers on one hand in the air.
- Cover one eye with the hand on that side.
- Cover an ear with the hand on that side.
- Touch a shoulder.
- Bend a knee.
- Put your hand on your hip.

Extending the Activity: The next time you perform this activity, do not do the movements with the children.

Observation and Evaluation: Does the child appropriately identify body parts? Is the child able to isolate one side from the other?

Adding Equipment: Some physical education suppliers offer vinyl cutouts of feet that are labeled right and left. Placing a pair of these in front of each child can help her or him see which side of the body is being used.

Curriculum Connectors: Positional concepts, like left and right, are a component of *mathematics* and *art*. Experimenting with the limitations and capabilities of body parts qualifies as *science*.

Let's Twist

♪ **"Twisting" (Length 2:10)—CD Track 19**

Unlike a turn, which rotates the whole body, a twist rotates a *part* of the body around an axis. It is perhaps through imagery that preschoolers and kindergartners can best relate to the nonlocomotor skill of twisting. With that in mind, ask them to twist in these ways:

- like the inside of a washing machine
- like a screwdriver when someone is using it
- like a wet dishrag being wrung
- as though wiping their bottoms with towels
- as though digging a little hole in the sand with a foot
- as though wiping with a towel and digging a little hole in the sand with a foot at the same time

Extending the Activity: Repeat the above activities, accompanying the movement with the song "Twisting." Also challenge children to discover how many body parts, besides the trunk, can twist. Possibilities include the arms, legs, and neck; the wrists, ankles, shoulders, and hips can twist to a lesser extent.

Observation and Evaluation: Does the child identify with the imagery used? Does the child differentiate between a twist and a turn?

Curriculum Connectors: Using the song incorporates *music*, while experimentation with the capabilities and limitations of body parts involves *science*. The self-expression required falls under the content area of *social studies*.

The Tightrope

This locomotor activity is an introduction to dynamic balance. To do this, you will need tightropes, whether imaginary or created.

Ask the children to pretend that they are tightrope walkers in the circus, balancing high above the crowd. You might want to remind them that there is a net below and that real tightrope walkers extend their arms to the sides for better balance.

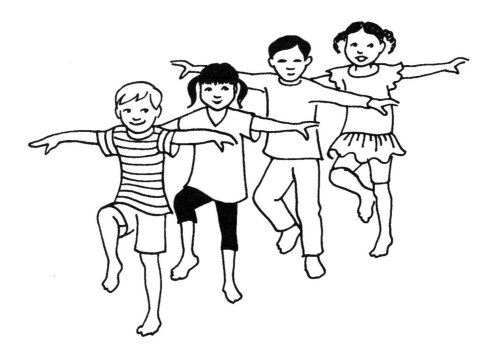

Extending the Activity: Once the children are able to move across the tightropes by walking in a forward direction, challenge them to find other locomotor skills they might use to travel across the tightropes. Then invite them to try moving sideways and finally backward on a tightrope.

Observation and Evaluation: Does the child use the arms for balance? Is the child placing one foot, heel to toe, in front of the other? Is the child able to maintain balance?

Adding Equipment: Most young children will find a visible tightrope much easier to walk on than an imaginary one. You can create tightropes by placing masking tape, yarn, or ropes on the floor. Make enough available so children do not have to wait long for a turn.

Curriculum Connectors: Balance is a component of *science*. Exploring the role of a tightrope walker (an occupation) falls under *social studies*. Directionality is critical to reading and writing (*language arts*).

Exploring Movement Elements

This activity uses locomotor skills that have already been introduced to the children with different elements of movement to vary the execution of these skills. The movement element being explored is cited in the second column.

Ask the children to do the following:

Movement	Movement Element
Walk in place.	space
Jump in a circle.	space
Run in place with knees high and arms low.	space and shape
Jump as hard as you can.	force
Walk as lightly as you can.	force
Jump-jump-stop; now repeat.	flow
Walk as slowly as you can.	time
Jump, making yourself as small as you can.	shape
Run, making yourself as tall as you can.	shape
Walk as quickly as you can.	time

Extending the Activity: You can make this activity more challenging by combining movement elements. For example, ask the children to do the following:

Movement	Movement Element
Walk backward while bending forward.	space and shape
Jump sideways as lightly as possible.	space and force
Run heavily, making yourself as tall as possible.	force and shape
Walk quickly, pausing every three steps.	time and flow

Observation and Evaluation: Does the child execute the locomotor skills correctly? Does the child vary the movement appropriately? Does the child respond appropriately when movement elements are combined?

Curriculum Connectors: Shape and spatial relationships are concepts central to *art*. Time is a component of *mathematics*, force and flow fall under the heading of *science*, and directionality is essential to reading and writing (*language arts*).

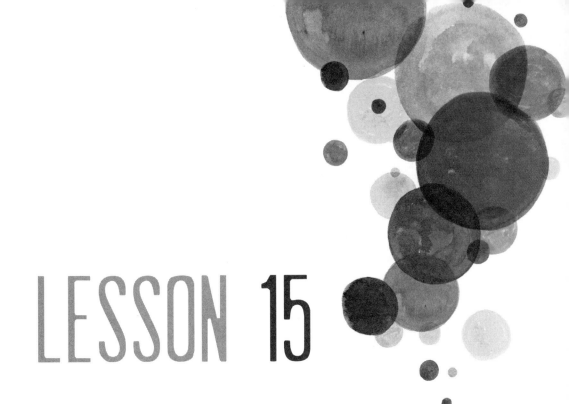

LESSON 15

Exploring Weight Placement

In this exercise, the children are going to experiment with the placement of weight on various body parts. You can explain the placement of weight by telling the children that only the body parts you assign will be touching the floor.

Ask them to place the following body parts on the floor:

- hands and knees only
- knees and elbows only
- knees alone
- just the tummy
- the back
- one side of the body; the other
- just the bottom
- hands and feet
- just the feet

Extending the Activity: Once children are familiar with this concept, add weight transferral to the activity. Explain that you want them first to put only those body parts you assign on the floor and then move to the next body parts assigned as *smoothly* as possible.

Observation and Evaluation: Is the child able to place his or her weight only on those body parts assigned? Can the child transfer weight smoothly from one position to the next?

Curriculum Connectors: Body-part identification, balance, and experimentation with weight placement and transferral qualify as *science* for young children.

In My Own Space

The chant below provides a review of various nonlocomotor skills. Challenge the children to first use the body as a whole and then to find different body parts capable of performing the skill.

The chant is as follows:

I can [nonlocomotor skill] my body,
Let me show you how.
There are parts that I can [same skill],
I'll show you those now.

Insert the following nonlocomotor skills where indicated in the chant above:

- bend
- swing
- shake
- bounce
- twist

Extending the Activity: When the children are ready, invite them to try the same process for other nonlocomotor skills.

Observation and Evaluation: Which nonlocomotor skills is the child able—or not able—to perform well? Is the child able to discover which body parts are capable of performing the various skills?

Curriculum Connectors: These activities provide experiences with *language arts* and, because of the body-part experimentation, *science*.

Let's Hop

A hop is a movement that propels the body upward from a takeoff on *one* foot. The landing is then made on the same foot, toe-ball-heel, with the knee bent. The free leg does not come in contact with the ground.

Demonstrate a hop to the children, and then ask them to show you hopping. You may find that some children have more success hopping in place, whereas others find it easier to hop around the room. If some children have trouble maintaining their balance, you might pair them up and ask them to hold hands, lift their outside legs, and hop together.

Extending the Activity: Children will first hop on the preferred foot. Once they have had ample experience with that, encourage them to try hopping on the nonpreferred foot. The next step is to invite them to hop around the room, changing feet often.

Observation and Evaluation: Is the child able to maintain balance? Does the child land with a bent knee, with the heel coming all the way to the floor? Can the child hop on both the preferred and nonpreferred foot?

Adding Equipment: Place one hoop per child on the floor, challenging the children to hop in and out, all the way around it. Also, place carpet squares or poly spots in a row on the floor, inviting the children to hop from one to the next. This can make hopping more fun for the children.

Curriculum Connectors: A discussion of gravity (the reason we cannot stay in the air when we hop) can link this activity to *science*, above and beyond the concept of balance involved.

Staccato/Legato

♪ **"Staccato/Legato" (Length 3:13)—CD Track 20**

This song offers experience with the musical elements of *staccato* and *legato* and the movement element of flow. Explain the two musical terms to the children. *Staccato* (stuh-CAH-toh) is short and separated notes and tends to inspire movement using a bound (interrupted) flow. *Legato* (lih-GAH-toh) is smooth and can be likened to free flow.

The form of the song is ABAB, with A representing staccato. Offer the following suggestions for movement:

Staccato	**Legato**
a robot moving	a butterfly floating
tiptoeing	ice skating
a stalking cat	an eagle soaring
a battery-operated toy	a weightless astronaut

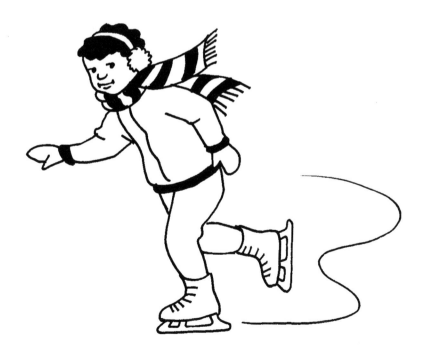

Extending the Activity: When repeating this activity, ask the children to simply show you how these two kinds of music make them feel like moving. You might also ask them to experiment with moving in the *opposite* way to each kind of music. Does it work?

Observation and Evaluation: Can the child differentiate between staccato and legato? Does the child move appropriately to each?

Adding Equipment: Make a variety of props available to the children, allowing them to choose which props work best for each section of the music. Possible props include streamers, ribbon sticks, maracas, hand drums, scarves, rhythm sticks, wooden blocks, and hoops.

Curriculum Connectors: Staccato and legato fall under the broader category of articulation in *music*. Active listening is central to *language arts*, and the self-expression required links the activity to *social studies*.

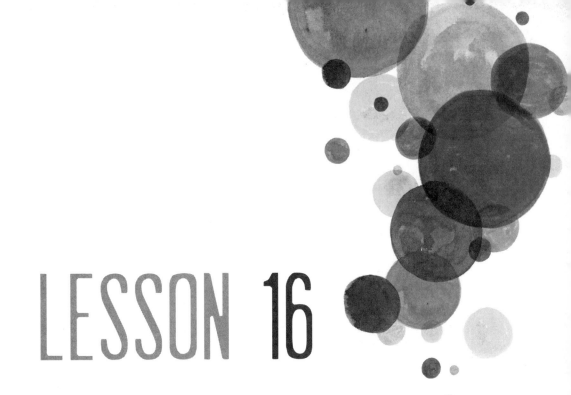

LESSON 16

Counting Body Parts

· ·

This exercise is similar to Exploring Weight Placement (page 136), in which you assigned body parts for the placement of weight. This time, however, you will simply give the children a *number* of body parts on which to place their weight, letting them choose the parts themselves.

Ask the children to place their weight on five, four, three, two, and one body part(s) at a time, challenging them to find at least two solutions to each combination (for example, a challenge to place weight on one part only could result in standing on the right or left foot, sitting on the bottom, or balancing on one or the other knee).

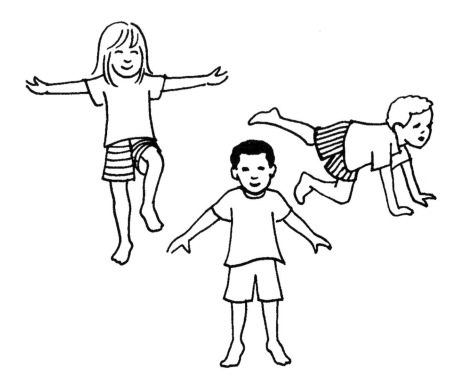

Extending the Activity: During repetitions of this activity, challenge the children to find *as many solutions as possible* to each combination. If necessary, remind them to try these challenges at low, middle, and high levels.

Observation and Evaluation: This is a simple way to assess whether or not the child is having difficulty with counting. Also, is the child able to find more than one solution to each challenge?

Curriculum Connectors: Counting, of course, is a component of *mathematics*. Because balance, stability, and body parts are also involved in these exercises, they offer experiences in *science* too.

Imitating Movement

This activity is similar to the Mirror Game (page 86), in which the children acted as your reflection as you performed a variety of movements one at a time. In this case, though, you will perform a short *sequence* of movements at a slow to moderate tempo, which the class must then imitate. An example would be this: bend knees—straighten—hands on hips.

Here are other possible sequences:

- rise on tiptoe—lower heels—clap hands twice
- bend forward at waist—straighten—hands on head
- jump twice in place—open and close mouth—shake arms

Extending the Activity: To make the activity more challenging, all you have to do is add to each sequence! Here are the same sequences, with two more steps added. Start by adding just one.

- bend knees—straighten—hands on hips—nod the head—circle arms
- rise on tiptoe—lower heels—clap hands twice—turn around—clap three times
- bend forward at waist—straighten—hands on head—jump once in place—blink three times
- jump twice in place—open and close mouth—shake arms—shake whole body—collapse to floor

Observation and Evaluation: Is the child able to replicate your sequence? If not, is it due to a problem remembering or in physically replicating what the eyes are seeing?

Curriculum Connectors: The ability to physically replicate what the eyes see is central to *language arts* (writing) and to *art*, while sequencing is a *mathematics* concept.

Let's Roll

A roll is generally defined as a movement made by a body that is *supine* (face up) or *prone* (face down) and fully extended, with the arms stretched overhead. Introduce the children to this type of roll, making sure they roll in both directions, both slowly and quickly.

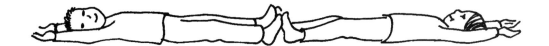

Extending the Activity: Once children are able to keep their bodies (and pathways) straight, ask them to try initiating the rolls with first the upper and then the lower torso. A more advanced activity is "footsie rolls," where children pair off, lying on their backs with the soles of their feet together. The object in this activity is for partners to roll over without their feet breaking contact. This one takes a lot of cooperation and enough room to move safely. For example, if you have a small area for movement, you may be limited to as few as one set of partners working at a time. Any waiting children can act as the audience, cheering or applauding while the partners remain connected and groaning when the connection is broken. Once the connection is broken, another pair takes a turn.

Observation and Evaluation: Is the child able to roll, in both directions, with a straight body? Can the child roll in a straight pathway? Does the child work cooperatively with a partner?

Curriculum Connectors: Rolling requires impetus (for example, a "jump start") and momentum, which are *science* concepts. Cooperative activities, of course, qualify as *social studies*.

Getting Fast/Getting Slow

♪ **"Getting Fast/Getting Slow" (Length 2:26)—CD Track 21**

Before beginning, explain the terms *accelerando* (ah-che-luh-RAHN-doh) and *ritardando* (rih-tar-DAHN-doh) to your students. Accelerando is music that gradually increases in tempo, whereas ritardando is music that gradually slows in tempo. The form of this song is ABAB, with A demonstrating accelerando.

Using a walk, lead the children around the room, increasing and decreasing your speed with the tempo of the music. If you find the children are having difficulty with this or they are becoming restless, feel free to call it quits after AB.

Extending the Activity: When the children are ready, let them take turns leading each other. Later you can challenge the children to move in any way they like to the increasing and decreasing tempo.

Observation and Evaluation: Can the child hear the increasing and decreasing tempo? Do the child's movements change accordingly?

Curriculum Connectors: Accelerando and ritardando are elements of *music* that go hand in hand with the movement element of time, which is a *mathematics* concept. Also, active listening is a component of *language arts*.

LESSON 17

Arms in Motion

. . . .

Ask the children to sit, and explain that they are going to experiment with how many ways they can move their arms alone. (*Note:* Because arms tire easily, you may have to include "resting" arms often.)

Have the children move both of their arms in the following ways:

- slowly
- quickly
- sharply
- swinging
- softly
- forcefully
- in a circular manner
- in straight lines

Extending the Activity: Challenge the children to move first the right (one) and then the left (the other) in the ways listed above. After they have had ample experience with this, ask them to move one arm in one of the ways listed above and then to move the other arm in the opposite way (for example, strongly and lightly; quickly and slowly).

You can also invite the children to play a game of Palm to Palm. In this partner activity, the children pair off and face each other, standing about a foot apart. The first child then places his or her arms into any position, with palms flat and facing the partner. The partner quickly places his or her palms against the first child's so they touch lightly. Once contact is made, the first child quickly assumes a new arm position, and the activity continues in this manner. After a while the partners reverse roles.

Observation and Evaluation: Is the child able to isolate the arms from the rest of the body? Can the child move the arms in the designated ways? Can the child isolate one arm from the other? Does the child work cooperatively with a partner? How creative is the child in finding arm positions? (If you find the arm positions all tend to be symmetrical, you might want to suggest that asymmetry is possible too; for example, one arm high and the other low.)

Adding Equipment: Holding a brightly colored scarf in each hand can make these activities more fun and visually appealing, and can also help children see the different responses better.

Curriculum Connectors: Because most of the ways in which you have asked the children to move their arms are descriptive words, these exercises (including the one exploring opposites) can be considered experiences in *language arts*. Palm to Palm, because it is an exploration of shape and is a cooperative activity, falls under the headings of *art* and *social studies*.

Let's Focus

This activity requires the children to isolate head movement and to use their imaginations to the maximum if they are to vary their responses.

Ask the children to focus their gaze as if doing the following:

- searching for something small in a rug
- looking out a car window
- trying to see in a dark room
- watching a falling star
- watching a parade
- being hypnotized by a swinging object
- looking through a telescope
- watching a tennis game
- looking at an airplane
- watching a race

Extending the Activity: With the children in pairs, one partner moves all around the room while the other remains stationary and maintains a constant focus on him or her. After a while, the partners reverse roles.

Observation and Evaluation: Does the child relate to the imagery used? Is the child able to concentrate to the extent required? Can the child isolate the head's movements from the rest of the body?

Curriculum Connectors: By focusing on the sense of sight, this activity qualifies as a *science* experience. The extension activity requires interaction and cooperation between partners, incorporating *social studies*.

Let's Slide

A slide is a gallop performed sideways, in which one foot leads and the other plays catch-up. The uneven rhythm remains the same as in the gallop. Facing forward, with feet together, the child slides one leg out to the side and then, with the weight primarily on that leg, slides the second leg in, so that the feet are once again together. The action, therefore, is step-close, step-close. Demonstrate the slide to the children and have them practice it to both sides.

Extending the Activity: When the children are ready, introduce some variations to the slide, remembering to have them slide to both the left and right side. For example, ask them if they can slide in these ways:

- quickly, then slowly
- lightly, then heavily
- in a circle
- with their arms out to the sides, then above their heads

Later, challenge them to form a circle, hold hands, and practice sliding in both directions. Ring Around the Rosie offers an opportunity to practice sliding.

Observation and Evaluation: Is the child able to face one direction and move in another? Does the child perform the slide with an uneven rhythm? Can the child slide in both directions?

Adding Equipment: Sliding is a locomotor skill commonly used to move a parachute in a circle. You might also want to beat out the correct rhythm on a hand drum, to add another sense to the experience, and especially to assist the auditory learners.

Curriculum Connectors: Accompanying the children's movements with a drum places greater emphasis on the rhythm, which is an element of *music*. Sliding as a group, because it is a cooperative activity, offers an experience in *social studies*.

Getting Louder/Getting Softer

♪ **"Getting Louder/Getting Softer" (Length 2:31)—CD Track 22**

This song will familiarize the children with the musical elements of *crescendo* (kruh-SHEN-doh) and *decrescendo* (day-kruh-SHEN-doh). Both musical terms refer to the volume of a musical passage. When there is a crescendo, the volume gradually gets louder. A decrescendo is just the opposite. The volume gradually gets softer. The form of the song "Getting Louder/Getting Softer" is ABAB, with A demonstrating crescendo and B demonstrating decrescendo.

Describe to the children what is going to happen with the music, and explain that they are going to use gentler movements when the music is soft and heavier movements when it is loud.

Begin by tiptoeing around the room with the children, either in a scattered formation or with them in line behind you, gradually increasing the weight of your steps as the music grows louder. By the time the volume is at its loudest, you should be stamping your feet. The music then begins to grow softer, as should your steps, until you are tiptoeing once again. You can end here if you feel the children need to stop, or you can repeat the sequence once again, ending with the song.

Extending the Activity: Challenge the children to move the way the music makes them feel like moving, reminding them that the music increases and decreases in volume and that their movements should increase and decrease in force correspondingly.

Once the children have ample experience with this, they can take partners and play the Shadow Game (page 117) to the accompaniment of this song. The challenge is for the leader to move appropriately to the music and for the "shadow" to match those movements. Halfway through the song, partners should reverse positions.

Observation and Evaluation: Can the child hear the gradually increasing and decreasing volume? Do the child's movements correspond to the music?

Curriculum Connectors: Crescendo and decrescendo are elements of *music* that go hand in hand with the movement element of force, involving light and heavy movements (light and heavy are quantitative concepts falling under *mathematics*). The partner activity, which requires cooperation, provides an experience in *social studies*, while physically replicating what the eyes are seeing is central to *art* and *language arts* (writing).

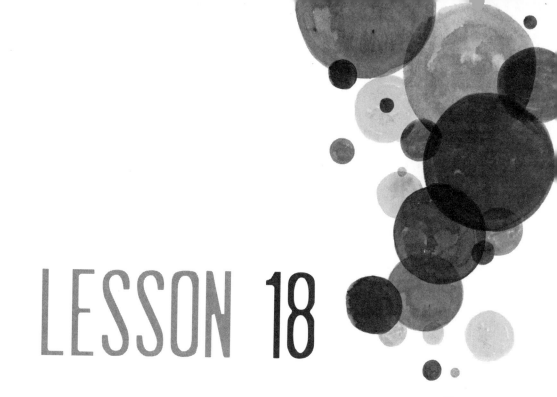

LESSON 18

Legs in Motion

In this activity, you will issue the same challenges presented in Arms in Motion (page 148), but the children will respond with their legs only. Therefore, they will have to be either sitting down or lying on their backs.

Have the children move their legs in the following ways:

slowly	softly
quickly	forcefully
sharply	in a circle
swinging back and forth	in straight lines

Extending the Activity: As you did with Arms in Motion, challenge the children to move first the right (one) leg and then the left (the other) leg in the ways listed above. After they have had ample experience with this, ask them to move one leg in one of the ways listed above and then to move the other leg in the opposite way (for example, strongly and lightly; quickly and slowly).

Observation and Evaluation: Is the child able to isolate the legs from the rest of the body? Can the child move the legs in the ways indicated? Can the child isolate one leg from the other?

Curriculum Connectors: The exploration of words for different types of movement, as well as opposites, constitutes *language arts*.

Pass a Movement

This activity depends upon group cooperation for its success.

Standing, form a circle with the children and begin by choosing an action that each child must imitate in her or his turn, until it comes back to you. For instance, you gently squeeze the hand of the child to your right, and he or she must do the same to the child to his or her right, and so on around the circle (sequential movement). Other simple actions follow:

- bending the knees and straightening
- stretching a leg
- jumping once
- hopping once
- bending at the waist and straightening
- raising and lowering arms

Extending the Activity: When the children are ready, let each of them have a turn choosing a movement to pass on.

Observation and Evaluation: Does the child understand the concept of sequential movement (that the movement is performed by only one person at a time, in turn)? Can the child replicate the movement passed? Is the child able to respond with an original movement?

Adding Equipment: You can certainly play this game using a prop. For example, the first child might demonstrate a movement with a beanbag. The movement and the beanbag are then passed to the next child, and so on around the circle.

Curriculum Connectors: The cooperative nature of this activity qualifies it as *social studies*, while sequence is a *mathematics* concept.

Let's Skip

. . . .

♪ "Skipping Song" (Length 1:09)—CD Track 23

A skip is actually a combination of two locomotor skills—a step and a hop. Like the gallop, a skip consists of an uneven rhythm. With more emphasis placed on the step than the hop, the overall effect becomes a light and skimming motion, during which the feet only momentarily lose contact with the ground.

Introduce skipping to the children, explaining that the skip is a combination of a step and a hop. There are many possibilities for teaching skipping, but you will most likely have to find a method that works with your particular group. Some children have learned to skip by pretending the floor was very hot, and that as soon as they stepped on it with one foot they would want to hop right back off it (and then repeat with the other foot). Some children may learn by imitation, and others learn by holding hands and skipping with someone who knows how. This latter method is particularly effective for children who can skip on one side and not the other (have them hold hands on the side on which they cannot skip).

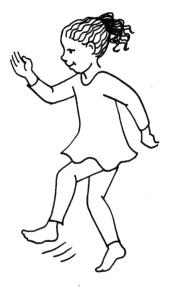

Extending the Activity: Play "Skipping Song" and ask the children to accompany it with skipping. Some children may find that the rhythm of the music helps. Once children are skipping successfully, provide some variety by suggesting they skip in circles, as lightly as possible, quickly, and in curving and zigzagging paths.

Observation and Evaluation: Is the child able to skip on both sides of the body? Does the child demonstrate the appropriate rhythm? Does the child use arms in opposition to the legs? Does the child maintain the proper posture?

Adding Equipment: Some children are aided in their quest to skip with vinyl cutout feet placed in a path on the floor.

Curriculum Connectors: In addition to the focus on rhythm, using the song provides experience with *music*. Rhythm and listening are essential components of both *music* and *language arts*.

Common Meters

♪ "Common Meters" (Length 3:59)—CD Track 24

This song is in four parts, performed in the common meters of 2/4, 3/4, 4/4, and 6/8. It is not important that the children understand the technical differences among the meters. What is important is that they be exposed to various meters and have the opportunity to physically experience them. So play the song, offering the following suggestions for how the children should move to each section:

- 2/4: clapping 1-2; stamping 1-2; marching; jumping
- 3/4: swaying; swinging arms; clapping 1-2-3; swinging a leg
- 4/4: clapping 1-2-3-4; running; nodding; conducting an orchestra
- 6/8: marching; clapping 1-2; moving head side to side; rocking

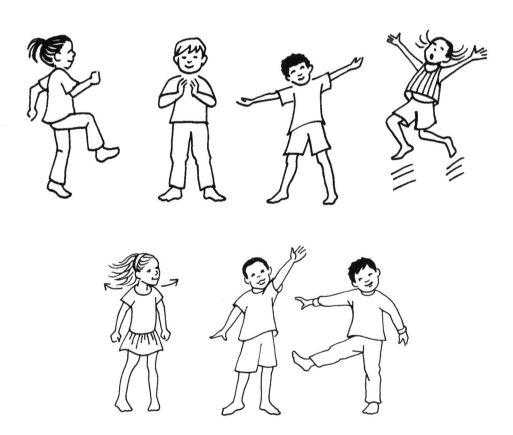

Extending the Activity: With repetitions of this activity, simply ask the children to move in whatever ways the music makes them feel. You can also challenge them to show you how the music makes the head, arms, hands, feet, or legs feel like moving.

Observation and Evaluation: Does the child differentiate among the meters? Do the child's movements change correspondingly?

Adding Equipment: You can provide children with handheld props, such as scarves, ribbon sticks, or streamers, and ask them to demonstrate how the music makes the prop feel like moving.

Curriculum Connectors: This activity is first and foremost an experience in *music*. However, if you choose to count the meters aloud, you can also add *mathematics* to the mix.

LESSON 19

Body-Halves Opposition

· ·

Asking separate halves of the body to perform opposite tasks is difficult for people of all ages, even when those tasks are not being performed at the same time. However, the children have had enough body and spatial awareness at this point to give it a try.

Have the children sit, and then explain that the right side of the body can do something separate from the left side, as can the top from the bottom. Then pose the following questions and challenges:

- Make a slow movement with one arm and then a fast movement with the other. (Now reverse sides.)
- Can you make a gentle, light movement with one arm and then a strong, hard movement with the other? (Now reverse.)
- Make a slow, light movement with your arms and hands, followed by a fast, hard movement with your legs and feet.

Extending the Activity: Additional challenges might include the following:

- Make your head move quickly, and then move one foot slowly.
- Can you make the other foot move fast and then your head move slowly?
- Stretch the top half of your body while also bending the lower half.

Observation and Evaluation: Does the child seem to understand the concept of body-halves opposition? Is the child capable of performing the tasks?

Curriculum Connectors: Experimentation with the limitations and capabilities of the body and its parts falls under the heading of *science* for young children. Also, discussion of and experience with opposites constitutes *language arts*.

Dodging in Place

A dodge generally involves the body as a whole as it moves quickly and forcefully to avoid an object moving toward it.

Using imagery to introduce the dodge to your preschoolers and kindergartners, ask them to pretend to dodge these things:

- a snowball
- a limb falling from a tree
- a flying Frisbee

Extending the Activity: You can make the activity more challenging by asking the children to imagine that they are dodging one snowball or tree limb after another, requiring them to dodge continuously.

Observation and Evaluation: Does the child move quickly and forcefully, as required by a dodge? Can the child identify with the imagery used?

Curriculum Connectors: Ask children to consider the change in the tension of their muscles when they dodge to incorporate *science*. The self-expression required in pretending qualifies as *social studies*.

Locomotion II

 "Locomotion II" (Length 4:47)—CD Track 25

This song is basically self-explanatory. Perform the verses nonmusically at first, with the children simply executing the locomotor skill called for in each. The lyrics are as follows:

Hey, everybody—look at me
And see what I can do.
I can walk so straight and tall,
And with good posture too!
Hey, everybody—look at me
And see what I can do.
I can run on my tiptoes,
And very quietly too!
Hey, everybody—look at me
And see what I can do.
I can hop on my right foot
And on my left one too!

Hey, everybody—look at me
And see what I can do.
I can skate as though on ice
And make you believe it too!
Hey, everybody—look at me
And see what I can do.
I can skip from here to there
And very lightly too!
Hey, everybody—look at me
And see what I can do.
I can sit in my own space
And wave good-bye to you!

Extending the Activity: Ask children what other locomotor skills they can perform, and create verses together to accompany them. When the children are familiar with the activity, add the song.

Observation and Evaluation: Is the child able to perform all the locomotor skills well? Which one could use more practice?

Curriculum Connectors: These activities provide experience with both *language arts* and *music*.

Different Strokes

· ·

♪ "Different Strokes" (Length 3:45)—CD Track 26

This song consists of four different styles: shuffle, Latin, waltz, and rock. Suggest the following ways of moving to each section:

- Style 1: Stepping in place; counting (and clapping) 1-2-3-4; bending and stretching; striking the air
- Style 2: Swaying the whole body or the head; turning right and left; swinging arms or legs; tiptoeing
- Style 3: Slow swaying; counting (and clapping) 1-2-3; taking slow and soft giant steps; slow stretches
- Style 4: Running; jumping; shaking; rolling

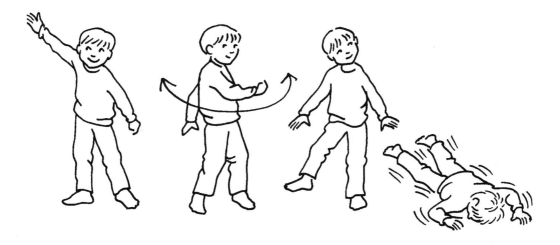

Extending the Activity: Invite the children to move in any way they want to the music. You can also play a game of Statues, in which the children move as long as the music is playing and then freeze into a statue when you pause the music.

Observation and Evaluation: Does the child differentiate among the styles? Does the movement change accordingly? Can the child improvise to music? While playing Statues, does the child demonstrate listening skills? Is the child able to stop and start on signal?

Adding Equipment: Make a variety of props available to the students, allowing them to choose the ones they feel are most appropriate for each style of music. Possible props include maracas, hand drums, streamers, ribbon sticks, tambourines, and rhythm sticks.

Curriculum Connectors: Style is an element of *music* that every child should experience. Listening skills are also a part of *language arts*. Stopping and starting on signal requires self-regulation skills, which fall under the content area of *social studies*.

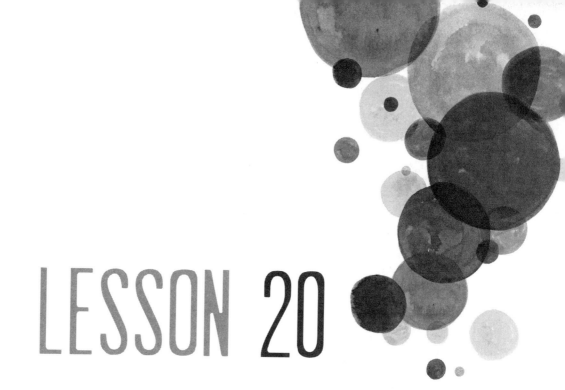

LESSON 20

Left Side/Right Side

· ·

This poem is an exercise in laterality, and you should initially perform it with the children, reminding them to perform their own actions, because this is not a mirroring activity. You will want to face them, though, which requires you to use the side opposite of what is called for in the poem. Remind them, too, that all responses are considered correct.

Read the poem out loud. The words are as follows:

There are many parts of the body
That come in twos, you know.
Like eyes and ears and hands and feet;
Shoulders, knees, and elbows.
And how do you tell one from the other
When they look just the same?
Well, one is right and one is left,
So now they have a name!
Your feet can take you to the right or left,
Heads can turn left to right.
Close one eye and not the other
And it will change your sight.
A turn can go to the right or left;
A hop can do the same.

Do you pitch with your left or right
When in a softball game?
It's not hard to kneel on your left knee
And bend your body right,
And show me on which side you lie
When you're in bed at night.
There are many, many other movements
You can do to either side.
Why don't you think of some others?
Your body is your guide!
Chorus: *Left side, right side,*
Show me if you can.
Left foot, right foot,
Right knee, right eye, left hand!

Extending the Activity: When the children are ready, challenge them to perform the activity without you.

Observation and Evaluation: Does the child know right from left? Does the child respond appropriately to the words?

Curriculum Connectors: In addition to experience with *language arts*, these activities provide practice with body-part identification, which comes under the heading of *science*.

Combining Nonlocomotor Skills

Having had a great deal of experience to this point with single nonlocomotor skills, the children should be ready to begin combining them. In this exercise, you will suggest combinations of nonlocomotor skills to the children, and they will put them together to form brief movement phrases. The children may perform as many repeats as they want of each individual skill, but they should link them without lengthy pauses or extraneous movements between them.

Suggest the following combinations to the children, and give them plenty of time to explore possibilities:

- bend-stretch-bend
- stretch-twist
- stretch-bend-swing
- sway-turn-sway
- sway-turn-shake

Extending the Activity: After ample experience with the preceding challenges, create longer sequences, such as the following:

- stretch-twist-swing-stretch
- sway-turn-sway-swing
- rock-dodge-shake-sit

You can also challenge the children to create their own combinations of nonlocomotor skills.

Observation and Evaluation: Is the child able to combine skills? Can the child remember the sequences after hearing them? Is the child able to perform all of the skills involved?

Curriculum Connectors: Creating movement phrases and sentences is similar to creating them in *language arts*.

Combining Locomotor Skills

In this exercise, you will suggest combinations of locomotor skills to the children, and they will put them together to form movement phrases. The children may perform as many repeats as they want of each skill, but they should link them without lengthy pauses or any extraneous movements between them.

Suggest the following combinations to the children:

- walk-hop-walk
- hop-run-hop
- run-leap-run
- run-jump-leap

Extending the Activity: After ample experience with the preceding challenges, create sequences using more challenging locomotor skills, such as the following:

- walk-hop-skip
- gallop-slide-leap
- jump-hop-leap

You can also challenge the children to create their own sequences of locomotor skills.

Observation and Evaluation: Is the child able to combine skills? Can the child remember the combinations after hearing them? Is the child able to perform all of the skills involved?

Curriculum Connectors: Creating movement phrases and sentences is similar to creating them in *language arts*.

Exploring Space

. . . .

🎵 **"Exploring Space" (Length 3:32)—CD Track 27**

This song is all about the movement element of space. If necessary, define what is meant by curving and zigzagging paths. Do the song nonmusically at first, asking the children to follow along with the lyrics, which are as follows:

Chorus: *It's easy to explore the space around you.*
C'mon, I will show you how.
First find a place to call your own,
Stand at your middle level now.

The verses then instruct the children to perform the following:

Reach high and bend low.
Take four steps forward and four backward.
Hop to the right and then to the left.
Make a curving and then a zigzagging path.
Finale: *It's easy to explore the space around you.*
You see, you have shown me how.
So find that place you call your own,
Relax at your middle level now.
Relax at your middle level now.

Extending the Activity: When the children are ready, add the song!

Observation and Evaluation: Does the child understand the instructions in the lyrics? Is the child able to successfully execute them?

Adding Equipment: Some children respond better to a *visible* personal space. You can provide each child with a carpet square, hoop, or poly spot to mark their "place they call their own."

Curriculum Connectors: In addition to experience with *language arts* and *music*, these activities are about the element of space, which is a component of both *mathematics* and *art*.

References

AAHPERD (American Alliance for Health, Physical Education, Recreation and Dance). 2009. *Active Start: A Statement of Physical Activity Guidelines for Children from Birth to Age 5.* 2nd ed. Reston, VA: AAHPERD.

Amabile, Teresa M. 1992. *Growing Up Creative: Nurturing a Lifetime of Creativity.* 2nd ed. Buffalo, NY: The Creative Education Foundation Press.

Bar-Or, Oded, John Foreyt, Claude Bouchard, Kelly D. Brownell, William H. Dietz, Eric Ravussin, Arline D. Salbe, Sandy Schwenger, Sachico St. Jeor, and Benjamin Torun. 1998. "Physical Activity, Genetic, and Nutritional Considerations in Childhood Weight Management." *Medicine and Science in Sports and Exercise* 30 (1): 2–10.

Carson, Linda M. 2001. "The 'I Am Learning' Curriculum: Developing a Movement Awareness in Young Children." *Teaching Elementary Physical Education* 12 (5): 9–13. Choosykids.com/CK2resources/eventhost/Day%202 /Body%20Language/The%201%20am%20Moving%20Curriculum.pdf.

CDC (Centers for Disease Control and Prevention). 2008. "Preventing Diabetes and Its Complications." http://www.cdc.gov/nccdphp/publications/factsheets /prevention/pdf/diabetes.pdf.

Frostig, Marianne. 1970. *Movement Education: Theory and Practice.* Chicago: Follett Education Corporation.

Gallahue, David L., and Frances Cleland Donnelly. 2003. *Developmental Physical Education for All Children.* 4th ed. Champaign, IL: Human Kinetics.

Graham, George. 2008. *Teaching Children Physical Education: Becoming a Master Teacher.* 3rd ed. Champaign, IL: Human Kinetics.

Halsey, Elizabeth, and Lorena Porter. 1970. "Movement Exploration." In *Selected Readings in Movement Education*, edited by Robert T. Sweeney, 71–77. Reading, MA: Addison-Wesley Publishing Company.

Hannaford, Carla. 2005. *Smart Moves: Why Learning Is Not All in Your Head.* 2nd ed. Salt Lake City, UT: Great River Books.

H'Doubler, Margaret Newell. 1925. *The Dance and Its Place in Education.* New York: Harcourt, Brace, and Company.

Kaur, Harsohena, Won S. Choi, Matthew S. Mayo, and Kari Jo Harris. 2003. "Duration of Television Watching Is Associated with Body Mass Index." *Journal of Pediatrics* 143 (4): 506–11. doi:10.1067/S0022-3476(03)00418-9.

Lewin, Tamar. 2010. "If Your Kids Are Awake, They're Probably Online." *New York Times*, January 20. http://www.nytimes.com/2010/01/20/education/20wired.html.

Mayesky, Mary. 2009. *Creative Activities for Young Children*. 9th ed. Clifton Park, NY: Delmar.

McDonough, Patricia. 2009. "Television and Beyond a Kid's Eye View." http://www.nielsen.com/us/en/newswire/2009/television-and-beyond-a-kids-eye-view.html.

Mosston, Muska, and Sara Ashworth. 1990. *The Spectrum of Teaching Styles: From Command to Discovery*. New York: Longman.

NAEYC (National Association for the Education of Young Children). 2009a. *Developmentally Appropriate Practice in Early Childhood Programs Serving Children from Birth through Age 8*. Position statement. Washington, DC: NAEYC. www.naeyc.org/files/naeyc/file/positions/PSDAP.pdf.

———. 2009b. *NAEYC Standards for Early Childhood Professional Preparation Programs*. Position statement. Washington, DC: NAEYC. http://www.naeyc.org/files/naeyc/file/positions/ProfPrepStandards09.pdf.

NIEER (National Institute for Early Education Research). 2010. "Preschool's Role in Fighting Childhood Obesity." *Preschool Matters* 8 (1): 12. http://nieer.org/sites/nieer/files/81.pdf.

Pate, Russell R., Kerry McIver, Marsha Dowda, William H. Brown, and Cheryl Addy. 2008. "Directly Observed Physical Activity Levels in Preschool Children." *Journal of School Health* 78 (8): 438–44. doi:10.1111/j.1746-1561.2008.00327.x.

Samuelson, Emily. 1981. "Group Development and Socialization through Movement." In *Readings: Developing Arts Programs for Handicapped Students*, edited by Lola H. Kearns, Mary Taylor Ditson, and Bernice Gottschalk Roehner, 53–54. Harrisburg, PA: Arts in Special Education Project of Pennsylvania.

Science Daily. 2010. "Obese Children Show Signs of Heart Disease Typically Seen in Middle-Aged Adults, Researcher Says." http://www.sciencedaily.com/releases/2010/10/101025005835.htm.

Sinclair, Caroline B. 1973. *Movement of the Young Child: Ages Two to Six*. Columbus, OH: Merrill.

Additional Resources

Sources for Ordering Musical Instruments

Childcraft
www.childcrafteducation.com
888-388-3224

Constructive Playthings
www.constructiveplaythings.com
800-448-1412

Lakeshore
www.lakeshorelearning.com
800-428-4414

MMB Music
www.mmbmusic.com
314-531-9635

Music in Motion
www.musicmotion.com
800-807-3520

Rhythm Band Instruments
www.rhythmband.com
800-424-4724

Sources for Ordering Equipment and Props

FlagHouse

www.flaghouse.com

800-793-7900

Kaplan Early Learning Company

www.kaplanco.com

800-334-2014

Lakeshore Learning

www.lakeshorelearning.com

800-428-4414

Play with a Purpose

www.pwaponline.com

888-330-1826

US Games

www.usgames.com

800-327-0484

About the Author

Rae Pica is an internationally recognized education consultant specializing in early childhood physical activity. Known for her lively and informative presentations and keynote speeches, she has also consulted for such groups as the *Sesame Street* Research Department, the Head Start Bureau, the Centers for Disease Control and Prevention, the President's Council on Physical Fitness and Sports, Nickelodeon's *Blue's Clues*, Mattel, and state health departments throughout the country. As founder and director of Moving & Learning (www .movingandlearning.com), Rae has been spreading the "movement message" since 1980.

Rae served on the original task force of the National Association for Sport and Physical Education that created *Active Start: A Statement of Physical Activity Guidelines for Children Birth to Age 5*. She is the author of eighteen books, including the three-book Moving & Learning series; *Physical Education for Young Children: Movement ABCs for the Little Ones*; *A Running Start: How Play, Physical Activity, and Free Time Create a Successful Child*, written for the parents of children ages birth to five; and the award-winning *Great Games for Young Children: Over 100 Games to Develop Self-Confidence, Problem-Solving Skills, and Cooperation* and *Jump into Literacy: Active Learning for Preschool Children*.

Additionally, Rae is cofounder of BAM! Radio Network (www.bamradionetwork .com), where she hosts the Internet radio programs *Teacher's Aid* and *Body, Mind, and Child*, and cohosts *NAEYC Radio*, interviewing experts in the fields of education, child development, play research, the neurosciences, and more.